UNIT 6

SUBSTANCE ABUSE PREVENTION ACTIVITIES

UNIT 6

SUBSTANCE ABUSE PREVENTION ACTIVITIES

PATRICIA RIZZO TONER

Just for the HEALTH of It!
Health Curriculum Activities Library

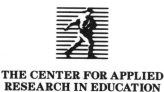

**THE CENTER FOR APPLIED
RESEARCH IN EDUCATION**
West Nyack, New York 10995

10 9 8 7 6 5 4 3

Library of Congress Cataloging-in-Publication Data

Toner, Patricia Rizzo, 1952-
    Substance abuse prevention activities / Patricia Rizzo Toner.
        p. cm.—(Just for the health of it! ; unit 6)
    "Includes 90 ready-to-use activities and worksheets for grades
7-12."
    ISBN 0-87628-879-4
    1. Substance abuse—Prevention—Study and teaching (Secondary)—
United States. I. Title. II. Series.
HV499.2.T66 1993
362.29'17'071273—dc20   93-14842
                                                              CIP

ISBN 0-87628-879-4

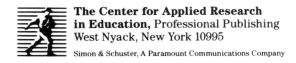
**The Center for Applied Research
in Education,** Professional Publishing
West Nyack, New York 10995
Simon & Schuster, A Paramount Communications Company

Printed in the United States of America

DEDICATION

To Third Lunch at Holland Junior High,
Council Rock School District
Holland, Pennsylvania

Dan Comisky, Mikki Grossman, Mitch Frank, Linda Deis, Colleen Leh,
Diane Wagner, Nancy Sides, Robin Hunt, Kathy Jesser, Bonnie Adler,
Donna Kokinda, Angela Felt, Marilyn Wasserman, Gloria Anderson,
Margaret Thatcher, Chris Simon, and assorted guests.

Thanks for all the laughter and fun we have shared over the years.
There is no need to abuse substances when we can spend a lunch period
abusing each other.

May you find peace and happiness in your lives.

Patricia R. Toner

ACKNOWLEDGMENTS

The source for some of the clip art images used in this resource is Presentation Task Force which is a registered trademark of New Vision Technologies Inc., copyright 1991.

Thanks to my son, Danny Toner, for walking the dog, feeding the cat, cleaning his room, taking out the trash, eating makeshift meals, and keeping me company while I spent countless hours typing and drawing.

Thanks to Sheila Murphy, Neshaminy School District, Langhorne, Pennsylvania, for the use of her Stages of Alcoholism game and her valuable suggestions.

Thanks to Colleen Leh for reading each activity and providing valuable feedback.

Thanks to the students in my Health classes for testing the materials and for providing honest feedback.

Thanks to Mike Flaherty, Holland Junior High, Holland, Pennsylvania, for being a supportive friend and colleague for the past 18 years.

Thanks to my mom and dad, Charles and Ruth Rizzo, Clementon, New Jersey, for providing us with an environment free of substance abuse as we grew up.

ABOUT THE AUTHOR

Patricia Rizzo Toner, M.Ed., has taught Health and Physical Education in the Council Rock School District, Holland, PA, for over 19 years, and she has also coached gymnastics and field hockey. She is the co-author of three books: *What Are We Doing in Gym Today?, You'll Never Guess What We Did in Gym Today!,* and *How to Survive Teaching Health.* Besides her work as a teacher, Pat is also a freelance cartoonist. A member of the American Alliance for Health, Physical Education, Recreation and Dance, Pat received the Hammond Service Award, the Marianna G. Packer Book Award and was named to *Who's Who Among Students in American Colleges and Universities,* as well as *Who's Who in American Education.*

ABOUT JUST FOR THE HEALTH OF IT!

Just for the Health of It! was developed to give you, the health teacher, new ways to present difficult-to-teach subjects and to spark your students' interest in day-to-day health classes. It includes over 540 ready-to-use activities organized for your teaching convenience into six separate, self-contained units focusing on six major areas of health education.

Each unit provides ninety classroom-tested activities printed in a full-page format and ready to be photocopied as many times as needed for student use. Many of the activities are illustrated with cartoon figures to enliven the material and help inject a touch of humor into the health curriculum.

The following briefly describes each of the six units in the series:

Unit 1: *Consumer Health and Safety Activities* helps students recognize advertising techniques, compare various products and claims, understand consumer rights, distinguish between safe and dangerous items, become familiar with safety rules, and more.

Unit 2: *Diet and Nutrition Activities* focuses on basic concepts and skills such as the four food groups, caloric balance or imbalance, the safety of diets, food additives, and vitamin deficiency diseases.

Unit 3: *Relationships and Communication Activities* explores topics such as family relationships, sibling rivalry, how to make friends, split-level communications, assertiveness and aggressiveness, dating, divorce, and popularity.

Unit 4: *Sex Education Activities* teaches about the male and female reproductive systems, various methods of contraception ranging from abstinence to mechanical and chemical methods, sexually transmitted diseases, the immune system, pregnancy, fetal development, childbirth, and more.

Unit 5: *Stress-Management and Self-Esteem Activities* examines the causes and signs of stress and teaches ways of coping with it. Along with these, the unit focuses on various elements of building self-esteem such as appearance, values, self-concept, success and confidence, personality, and character traits.

Unit 6: *Substance Abuse Prevention Activities* deals with the use and abuse of tobacco, alcohol, and other drugs and examines habits ranging from occasional use to addiction. It also promotes alternatives to drug use by examining peer pressure situations, decision-making, and where to seek help.

To help you mix and match activities from the series with ease, all of the activities in each unit are designated with two letters to represent each resource as follows: Sex Education (SE), Substance Abuse Prevention (SA), Relationships and Communication (RC), Stress Management and Self-Esteem (SM), Diet and Nutrition (DN), and Consumer Health and Safety (CH).

About Unit 6

Substance Abuse Prevention Activities, Unit 6 in *Just for the Health of It!,* gives you ninety ready-to-use activities to develop your students' awareness of the effects and dangers inherent in the use of tobacco, alcohol, and other drugs. The activities include reproducibles to hand out to students, innovative games, puzzles, and other techniques to enhance your presentations.

You can use these aids in any way you wish—to introduce a particular subject, to heighten students' interest at any given point in a lesson, or to reinforce what students have already learned. Complete answer keys for the activity sheets are provided at the end of the unit. You may keep these for your own use or place a copy at some central location for student self-checking.

For quick selection of appropriate activities, the table of contents provides general and specific topic heads and a complete listing of all worksheets and other activities in the unit. The ninety activities are organized into four main sections, including:

Alcohol. The twenty-three reproducibles and activities in this section help students learn about the dangers of alcohol and the identifying factors of addiction. Some of the main topics are:
- Alcohol's Effect on the Body
- Understanding Addiction to Alcohol
- Stages of Alcoholism

Smoking. This section offers more than twenty-five activities focusing on these and other topics:
- Chemicals in Cigarette Smoke
- Research on Lung Diseases
- Anti-smoking Activities

Drugs. Over twenty-five reproducibles and activities in this section cover topics such as:
- Understanding Methods and Types of Drugs
- Profiles of Drugs
- Types of Drug Abuse

General Activities. The fourth main section features additional supplementary activities ranging from "Advertising Techniques that Promote the Use of Drugs" to "Legal Consequences of Drug Use" and a "Substance Abuse Jeopardy Game."

All of the reproducibles and activities in this unit are numbered consecutively and keyed to the unit with the letters **SA,** representing the Substance Abuse Prevention component of the series. These worksheets, games, puzzles, and activities can be put directly into your lessons.

I hope you'll enjoy using them as much as I do.

Patricia Rizzo Toner

CONTENTS

SMOKING   27

What Do You Know About Smoking?

Chemicals in Cigarette Smoke

Research on Lung Disease

Smoking Vocabulary Matching Game

ALCOHOL

- **What Do You Know About Alcohol?**

- **Alcohol's Effect on the Body**

- **Considering Other Effects of Alcohol**

- **Understanding Addiction to Alcohol**

- **Stages of Alcoholism**

ALCOHOL PRE-TEST (SA-1)

DIRECTIONS: Place a *T* for True or an *F* for False in the blank to the left.

_____ 1. Beer is "weaker" than rum or vodka.

_____ 2. Alcohol is digested the same way food is digested in the body.

_____ 3. Because alcohol is a stimulant, it tends to pep you up.

_____ 4. The liver is the organ responsible for "burning up" the alcohol in the body.

_____ 5. The body can eliminate about 5 ounces of alcohol per hour.

_____ 6. BAC or BAL refers to the amount of calories in an alcoholic beverage.

_____ 7. Black coffee and a cold shower can help to sober you up.

_____ 8. It is possible to die from an overdose of alcohol.

_____ 9. Alcohol does the greatest damage to the liver, brain, and heart.

_____ 10. Alcohol is high in calories and has no nutritional value.

©1993 by The Center for Applied Research in Education

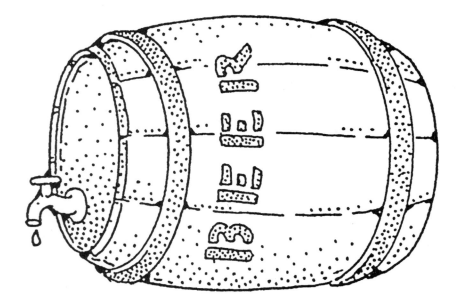

WHAT'S IN A DRINK? (SA-2)

DIRECTIONS: Find out the percentage of alcohol, plus the other ingredients in the beverages below and place the information in the blanks. Remember: a 5 oz. glass of wine, a 12 oz. can of beer and a 1½ oz. shot of hard liquor all have the same amount of alcohol.

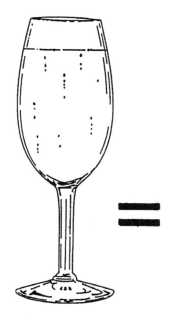
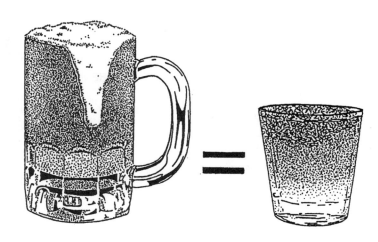

| 5 oz. of wine has ½ oz. alcohol | = | 1 can (12 oz.) beer has ½ oz. alcohol | = | 1 ½ oz. shot has ½ oz. alcohol |

INGREDIENTS:

Beer: _____ % of alcohol, plus _____

_____

_____

Wine: _____ % of alcohol, plus _____

_____

_____

Hard Liquor: _____ % of alcohol, plus_____

_____

_____

PROOF IT!! (SA-3)

Proof indicates the concentration of alcohol in a beverage. The amount of alcohol is determined by dividing the proof number in half. The higher the proof, the stronger the alcohol.

DIRECTIONS: Place the PROOF or PERCENTAGE in the blank.

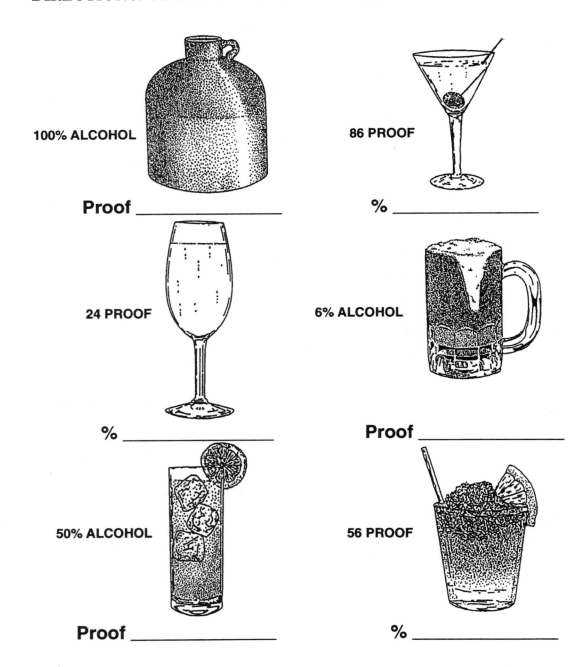

100% ALCOHOL

Proof _____

86 PROOF

% _____

24 PROOF

% _____

6% ALCOHOL

Proof _____

50% ALCOHOL

Proof _____

56 PROOF

% _____

THE PATH OF ALCOHOL (SA-4)

5. BRAIN. Alcohol goes to the brain almost as soon as it is consumed. The alcohol keeps passing through the brain until the liver has had a chance to oxidize it (burn it up).

1. MOUTH. Alcohol is consumed and passes down the esophagus.

4. BLOODSTREAM. The heart pumps the blood (and the alcohol) to all parts of the body.

6. LIVER. The liver burns up or oxidizes the alcohol at the rate of ½ ounce per hour. This process of oxidation is when the liver changes alcohol into water, carbon dioxide, and energy. The body then eliminates the water by sweating and urinating, and the carbon dioxide by breathing. This is why it is possible to smell alcohol on the breath of a person who has been drinking.

2. STOMACH. A little alcohol goes through the stomach walls and into the bloodstream, but most passes into the small intestines.

3. SMALL INTESTINES. Alcohol is rapidly absorbed through the walls of the small intestines and into the bloodstream.

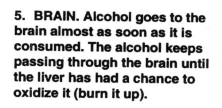

THE EFFECT OF ALCOHOL ON THE BRAIN (SA-5)

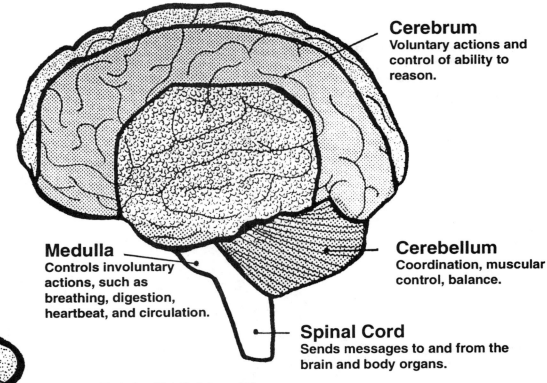

Cerebrum
Voluntary actions and control of ability to reason.

Medulla
Controls involuntary actions, such as breathing, digestion, heartbeat, and circulation.

Cerebellum
Coordination, muscular control, balance.

Spinal Cord
Sends messages to and from the brain and body organs.

©1993 by The Center for Applied Research in Education

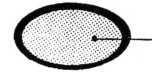

1 to 2 Drinks (BAC .01 to .05)

Person's systems begin to slow down, relaxed feeling, less inhibited, slight decrease in fine motor skills. Person should wait at least an hour before driving.

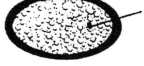

3 to 4 Drinks (BAC .05 to .10)

Fine motor skills are decreased, performance and responsiveness are reduced. There is a reduction in judgment as well as reaction time. People may feel more alert and talkative, but, in reality, the systems are slowed.

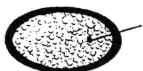

5 to 7 Drinks (BAC .10 to .18)

The senses are dulled, especially speech, hearing, and vision. Balance is altered and person may stagger. There is a decreased sense of pain.

8 to 12 Drinks (BAC .20 to .33)

The reflex actions are decreased, body temperature drops, blood circulation slows, as does respiration. Unconsciousness may occur. Further drinking may cause coma and eventual death from alcohol overdose.

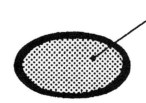

NOTE: These blood alcohol concentrations (BACs) are based on a 130 lb. person who has consumed the alcohol in a 1- to 2-hour span of time.

DRUNK DRIVING CHART (SA-6)

DIRECTIONS: The liver can oxidize or burn up approximately ½ ounce of alcohol per hour. Nothing can speed up this process. Remember, it is always best to wait at least one hour per drink before driving...or let someone who hasn't been drinking drive. Color the chart below green, yellow, and red, as indicated.

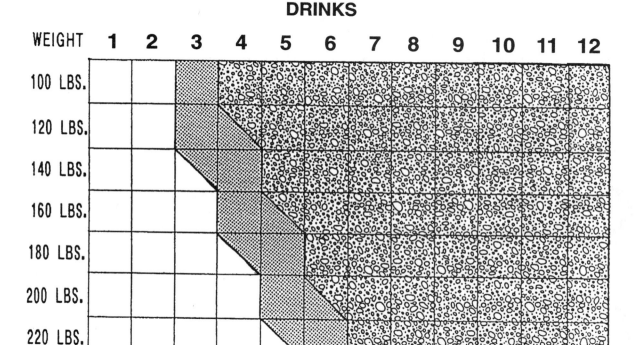

DRINKS

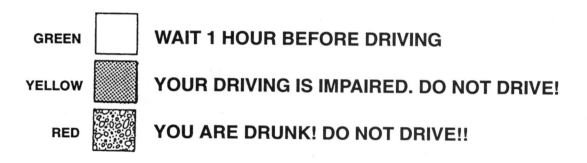

GREEN — WAIT 1 HOUR BEFORE DRIVING

YELLOW — YOUR DRIVING IS IMPAIRED. DO NOT DRIVE!

RED — YOU ARE DRUNK! DO NOT DRIVE!!

7

ACTIVITY 1: BULLETIN BORED?

Concept/ Description: Every day people are affected by alcohol-related thefts, accidents, and fights.

Objective: To show students that there are many alcohol-related problems in their own community.

Materials: Bulletin board space
Local newspapers from different days
Construction paper, scissors
Stapler, staples

Directions:
1. Have students cut out every article in the local newspaper relating to alcohol. Articles could include police logs and drunk-driving accident reports.
2. Place all the articles on the bulletin board.
3. Have students come up with an appropriate heading or theme and cut the letters out of construction paper.
4. Examples of headings are: Drink, Drive, Die! or Drinking and Driving Could KILL a Friendship!

Variation: Have students write essays, design posters, or write poems about the abuse of alcohol and add them to the bulletin board.

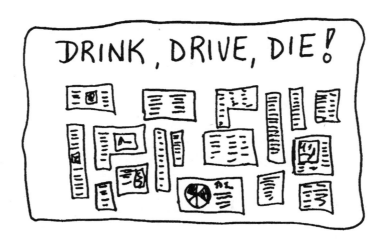

©1993 by The Center for Applied Research in Education

Name _____ Date _____

YOU BE THE JUDGE!! (SA-7)

DIRECTIONS: Listed below are some situations involving alcohol. Decide if each action described is legal or illegal and write your decision in the blank. Find out the drinking laws for your state (contact the local police department) and check your answers.

1. A 6-year-old boy has a sip of his grandfather's beer at a family barbecue.

2. A junior high school student buys a few wine coolers. _____

3. Your parents puchase a wine-making kit and make a few bottles of wine. _____

4. A high school student wears a T-shirt promoting beer drinking. _____

5. A 30-year-old woman buys a six-pack of beer from a bar on a Sunday. _____

6. A 21-year-old lends his 16-year-old brother his driver's license so he can buy alcohol. _____

7. A 15-year-old girl is at a drinking party that is raided by the police. She has an open can of beer in her hand but she has not had a drink. _____

8. A 22-year-old college student has a few beers at a local bar and hits a tree while driving home. His BAC is .04 percent. Is his blood-alcohol level legal or illegal? _____

9. A drunken man starts a fight at a movie theater and pushes a patron to the ground. _____

10. A waiter serves a glass of champagne to a 17-year-old who is celebrating her birthday with her parents. _____

11. A high school student "spikes" the punch at a school dance. _____

12. A woman drives home from a party and is stopped by the police for weaving all over the road. She refuses to take a breathalyzer test. _____

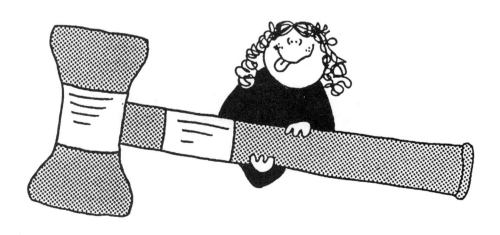

ALCOHOL CROSSWORD PUZZLE (SA-8)

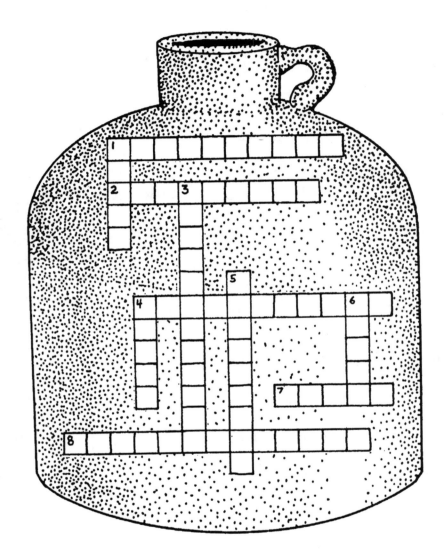

©1993 by The Center for Applied Research in Education

DOWN

1. Two times the percentage of alcohol in a beverage.
3. Process by which alcohol enters the bloodstream and travels to all body parts.
4. The type of alcohol used in beverages.
5. Liver disease caused by drinking heavily for many years.
6. The liver can burn up ½ _____ of alcohol per hour.

ACROSS

1. One-half of the proof.
2. Process by which the liver burns up the alcohol consumed.
4. Process by which the alcohol leaves the body.
7. Organ responsible for oxidizing alcohol.
8. During oxidation, the alcohol is changed to water, energy, and _____ (2 wds).

Name _____   **Date** _____

EFFECTS OF ALCOHOL (SA-9)

DIRECTIONS: Fill in the blanks to explain how alcohol affects a person.

HOW ALCOHOL AFFECTS A PERSON DEPENDS ON:

1. How _____ you drink.

2. How _____ you drink.

3. Your body_____.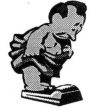

4. How much drinking you've done in the _____.   **I've been drinking for 5 years now!**

5. How much _____ is in the stomach.

6. What your _____ are about drinking.   **I'm gonna get loaded!!**

7. _____ you are when you drink.    **PARTY**

Name _____ **Date** _____

REASONS TO DRINK

REASONS TO ABSTAIN (SA-10)

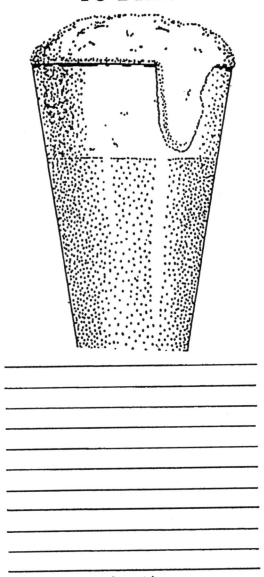

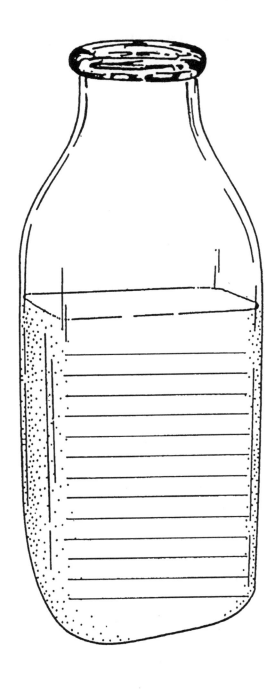

DIRECTIONS: On the lines provided, list all the reasons you can think of for underage drinking. Next list all the reasons you can think of for *not* drinking (abstaining).

EXPLODING THE MYTHS (SA-11)

DIRECTIONS: Numbered below are six myths about drinking. Below them are six correct explanations that "explode" or disprove each myth. Match each myth with its correct explanation by placing a number in the box.

1 It's OK to drive if you've only had a few drinks.

2 Drinking black coffee can sober you up.

3 Mixing drinks will make you drunker.

4 Drink milk before drinking to coat the stomach and you won't get as drunk.

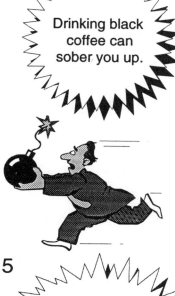

5 All alcoholics are skid row bums.

6 Taking a cold shower can sober you up.

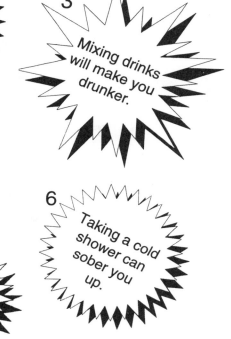

☐ WRONG. The only thing you'll be is wet. Showers cannot sober you up.

☐ WRONG. Drinking black coffee will make you no less drunk. Time is the only thing that can sober you up. You'll only be a wide-awake drunk.

☐ WRONG. Anyone can become an alcoholic. You can be young or old, rich or poor, any race or religion.

☐ WRONG. Mixing drinks may make you ill, but it's the amount that you drink that makes you drunk, not the flavor.

☐ WRONG. Even a couple of drinks can impair judgement, reaction time, vision, etc.

☐ WRONG. Milk and all other foods may slow down alcohol's effects, but the alcohol will still get into your bloodstream.

ACTIVITY 2 : TV TIME
(Alcohol's Target Audiences)

Concept/
Description: Advertisers carefully plan the type of ads to be shown and the time they are to be aired so as to target particular audiences.

Objective: To have students understand that since alcohol is a product that kills people, it is necessary for the alcohol industry to recruit new users every day. The main method of reaching potential users is through television.

Materials: TV Time Worksheet (SA-12)
TV Time Sign-Up Sheet (SA-13)

Directions:
1. Have each student sign up for a half-hour time slot to watch TV at some point during the week.
2. Each student receives a TV Time Worksheet and answers the questions while watching TV during their allotted time slot.
3. Remind students to be especially aware of the alcohol ads shown during that half-hour time period.
4. Discuss the students' findings and compile the results. When were the most alcohol-related ads shown? What types of ads were shown during sports events? To whom do the ads seem to be geared in each case, etc.?
5. Since the alcohol industry sells a product that can kill people (approximately 400 people die per week in alcohol-related auto accidents), where do the students think the "replacement" drinkers come from? Discuss.
6. Have students give examples of alcohol ads that are geared toward younger drinkers (the former Spuds MacKenzie, the Swedish Bikini Team, etc.).

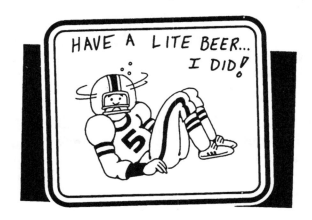

Name _____ **Date** _____

TV TIME WORKSHEET (SA-12)

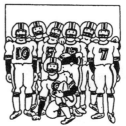

Name _____

TV Time Slot _____

Day of Week _____

Channel Watched _____

Program Watched _____

Number of Alcohol Ads (use slash marks / / / /) _____

Alcohol Ad Analysis

Product	Time Shown	General Description	Length	Target Audience
Bud Light	8:13	Playing beach volleyball.	30 sec.	men teenagers

Comments/Reaction:

Name _____   Date _____

TV TIME SIGN-UP SHEET (SA-13)

TIME	M	T	W	R	F	SA	SU
4:00–4:30							
4:30–5:00							
5:00–5:30							
5:30–6:00							
6:00–6:30							
6:30–7:00							
7:00–7:30							
7:30–8:00							
8:00–8:30							
8:30–9:00							
9:00–9:30							
9:30–10:00							

HOW MUCH DO YOU KNOW? (SA-14)

ADDICTION

DIRECTIONS: Place a *T* for True or an *F* for False in the blank to the left of each statement.

_____ 1. Abuse of alcohol can lead to addiction.

_____ 2. Use of alcohol and other drugs becomes the most important thing in a person's life once they are addicted.

_____ 3. Alcoholism is not a disease.

_____ 4. Anyone who drinks is likely to have an alcohol problem.

_____ 5. After an addict has successfully stopped "using," he or she can never use alcohol or other drugs again.

_____ 6. The brain and liver suffer the most damage when a person drinks heavily for many years.

_____ 7. There are signs to warn a person that his or her "using" may be leading to addiction.

_____ 8. When a person uses alcohol or other drugs for a long period of time, tolerance develops causing the person to need more of the substance to feel "high."

_____ 9. Unpleasant physical and emotional symptoms occur when an addict tries to stop using the substance to which they are addicted.

_____ 10. Drinking or using drugs when alone is a warning sign that may indicate addiction.

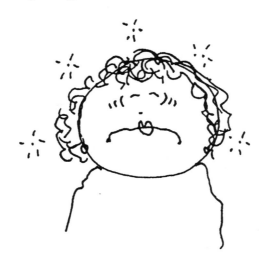

CHECKLIST– ADDICTION (SA-15)

DIRECTIONS: Check as many boxes as apply to you or someone you know.

DO YOU OR DOES SOMEONE YOU KNOW...

☐ 1. spend a great deal of time talking or thinking about getting "high"?

☐ 2. use drugs or alcohol when alone or when no one else is using?

☐ 3. have a "blackout" or memory loss during or after a drinking or drugging episode?

☐ 4. hoard or protect an extra supply of drugs or alcohol so as not to run out?

☐ 5. need more and more of a substance to get the desired effect?

☐ 6. drink more or use more drugs than originally planned or do so without planning?

☐ 7. use alcohol or drugs to escape from problems?

☐ 8. chug or gulp drinks, take large amounts of drugs, or do anything to get a large amount of a substance into the body quickly?

☐ 9. find that "using" is upsetting or worrying the family?

☐ 10. appear less efficient or ambitious?

☐ 11. lose time from school or work due to alcohol or drug use?

☐ 12. need to drink or use drugs first thing in the morning?

If you have checked even some of these boxes, it may indicate a drug or alcohol problem. You or the person you know may need help. Ask your teacher or counselor to advise you as to the best source of help in your area.

ACTIVITY 3 : PAGES OF STAGES
(Stages of Alcoholism)

Concept/ Description: Alcoholism is a chronic, progressive, and potentially fatal disease.

Objective: To have students understand the progression of the disease of alcoholism.

Materials: The Stages of Alcoholism Cards (SA-17 to SA-21)
Scissors
Wall Space, large sheets of oaktag, or space on the floor
Tape

Directions:
1. Divide the class into groups of three or four students.
2. Give each group a Stages of Alcoholism sheet and ask them to cut out the squares.
3. Ask each group to put the cards into three categories: Early Stages, Middle Stages, and Final Stages. This can be done in a number of ways:
   a. Tape each card to three areas on the wall.
   b. Tape each card to three separate sheets of oaktag or construction paper.
   c. Place the cards in three piles on the floor.
   d. Tape the cards to three areas on the chalkboard.
4. After each group is finished, give the correct answers and discuss.
5. Ask if the students are surprised to find that memory blackouts occur in the early stages, or if they realized that as the disease progresses it becomes more and more difficult to get "high" no matter how much is consumed.

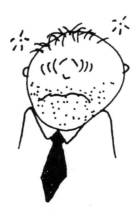

STAGES OF ALCOHOLISM (SA-16)

Early

Makes promises to quit and can't keep them

Drinks often to relieve tension

Increased tolerance (need more and more to feel the effects)

Personality changes

Memory blackouts

More forgetful

More irritable

Middle

Tries to deny or hide drinking

Drinks when alone

Drinks in the morning

Signs of drinking more noticeable

Drinks at work or at school

Harder to feel "high" no matter how much consumed

Drinking a daily necessity

Final

Isolation from friends

Isolation from family

Loneliness

Lives to drink

Never seems to eat

Nervous

Takes vitamins and tranquilizers, but neither helps

Very tense

Very irritable

Liquor more important than family or job

Tremors (shakes)

Hallucinations

Weakness due to malnutrition

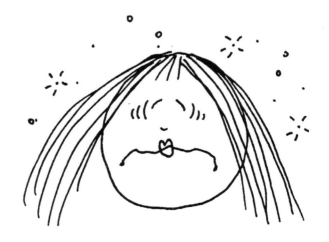

STAGES OF ALCOHOLISM CARDS (SA-17)

Never seems to eat	**Liquor more important than family or job**
Nervous	**Takes vitamins and tranquilizers, but neither helps**
Memory blackouts	**Drinking a daily necessity**
Very irritable	**Very tense**

STAGES OF ALCOHOLISM CARDS (SA-18)

Harder to feel "high" no matter how much consumed

Drinks in the morning

Signs of drinking more noticeable

Personality changes

Tremors (shakes)

Drinks at work or at school

Loneliness

Hallucinations

STAGES OF ALCOHOLISM CARDS (SA-19)

Makes promises to quit and can't keep them	**More irritable**
Weakness due to malnutrition	**More forgetful**
Tries to deny or hide drinking	**Isolation from friends**
Drinks when alone	**Lives to drink**

STAGES OF ALCOHOLISM CARDS (SA-20)

Increased tolerance	**Drinks often to relieve tension**
Isolation from family	

MAKE YOUR OWN CARDS (SA-21)

SMOKING

- **What Do You Know About Smoking?**

- **Chemicals in Cigarette Smoke**

- **Research on Lung Diseases**

- **Smoking Vocabulary Matching Game**

- **Legal Consequences Regarding Smoking**

- **Anti-Smoking Activities**

Name _____ Date _____

TEST YOUR SMOKING I.Q. (SA-22)

DIRECTIONS: Place a *T* for True or an *F* for False in the blank to the left.

_____ 1. The nicotine in cigarettes causes cancer.

_____ 2. The tar in cigarettes causes addiction.

_____ 3. Cigarette smoking can lead to heart disease.

_____ 4. Over 1,000 people die each day from smoking.

_____ 5. It is safe to smoke filtered cigarettes.

_____ 6. Chewing tobacco contains less nicotine than cigarettes.

_____ 7. Nine out of ten people with lung cancer will die.

_____ 8. Being in a smoke-filled room for one hour is the same as smoking one cigarette.

_____ 9. A woman who smokes during pregnancy can harm the fetus.

_____ 10. Polonium is a radioactive element found in cigarette smoke.

_____ 11. Cigarette smoking kills more people each year than all the deaths due to AIDS, heroin, crack, cocaine, car accidents, murder, fire, and alcohol combined.

_____ 12. Smoking pipes and cigars is a great deal less dangerous than smoking cigarettes.

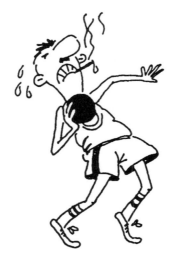

Name _____   Date _____

SMOKE 'N CROAK! (SA-23)

DIRECTIONS : Cigarette smoking kills more than 350,000 Americans each year. Unscramble the words and fill them into the sentence below to find out an important fact about deaths due to cigarette smoking.

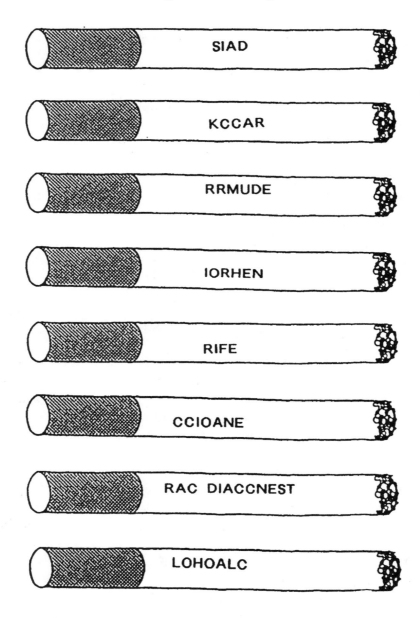

SIAD

KCCAR

RRMUDE

IORHEN

RIFE

CCIOANE

RAC DIACCNEST

LOHOALC

Cigarette smoking kills more people per year than all the deaths due to _____ , _____ ,

_____ , _____ , _____ , _____ , _____ , & _____ combined!

ACTIVITY 4 : SMOKE GETS IN YOUR LUNGS
(Chemicals in Cigarette Smoke)

Concept/ Description: There are more than 3,000 harmful chemicals present in tobacco smoke.

Objective: Students will see the types of chemicals to which the lungs are exposed if a person chooses to smoke.

Materials: Smoke Gets in Your Lungs Worksheet (SA-24)
Up in Smoke! Worksheet (SA-25)
Scissors
Glue

Directions:
1. Pass out the Smoke Gets in Your Lungs worksheet, and the Up in Smoke! worksheet.
2. Have students cut the names of the chemicals out and glue them onto the picture of the lungs.
3. Discuss the harmfulness of these chemicals and ask students why people would still continue to smoke knowing that they are damaging their bodies.

Variations:
1. Have students write the chemical names onto the picture of the lungs rather than cut and paste.
2. Have an anti-smoking slogan contest. Put the best slogan together with the diagram of the lungs containing the names of the chemicals and send the diagram to a printer to have T-shirts made. Perhaps the PTO would be willing to sponsor the activity.

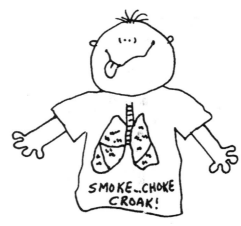

SMOKE GETS IN YOUR LUNGS (SA-24)

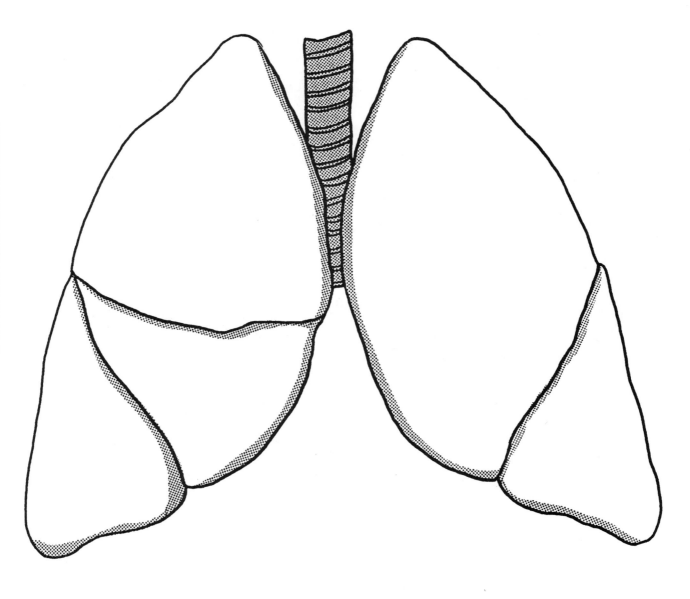

UP IN SMOKE! (SA-25)

DIRECTIONS: Listed below in the "cloud of smoke" are some of the more than 3,000 chemicals found in cigarette smoke. Research any five chemicals and find out what other products contain the chemicals you select. Place your answers on the Up in Smoke Research Sheet. (SA-26)

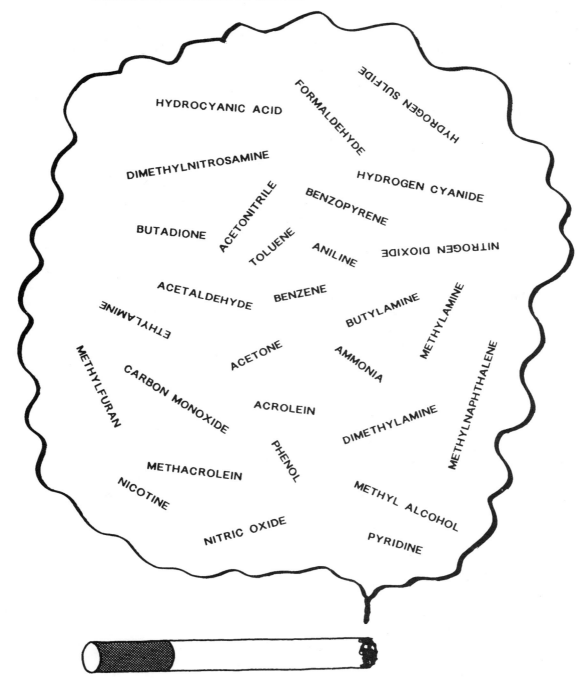

UP IN SMOKE! (SA-26)

Acetone	nail polish remover paint thinner brush cleaner paint remover
1	
2	
3	
4	
5	

WHAT SMOKING CAN DO FOR YOU: (SA-27)

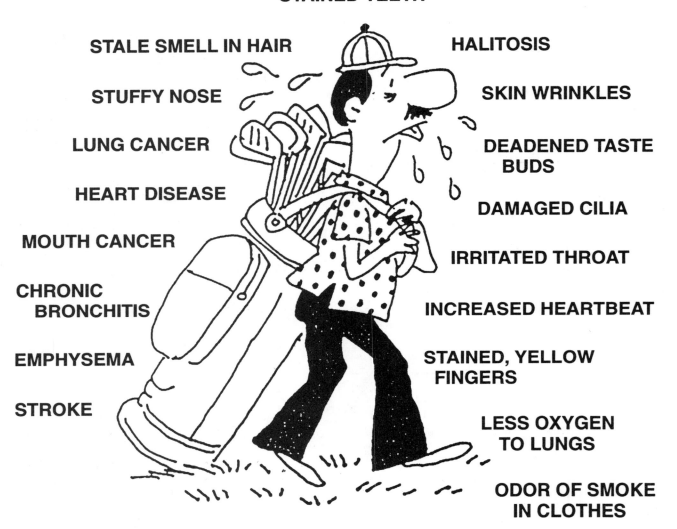

SMOKING KILLS OVER 1,000 PEOPLE EACH DAY!

WHAT CHEWING TOBACCO CAN DO FOR YOU: (SA-28)

MOUTH SORES

CANCER OF THE:

CHEEK
MOUTH
TONGUE
LIPS

INCREASE YOUR RISK OF:

PHARANGEAL CANCER
ESOPHAGEAL CANCER

HALITOSIS (BAD BREATH)

LIP STAINS

DISCOLORED TEETH

DESTRUCTION OF GUMS

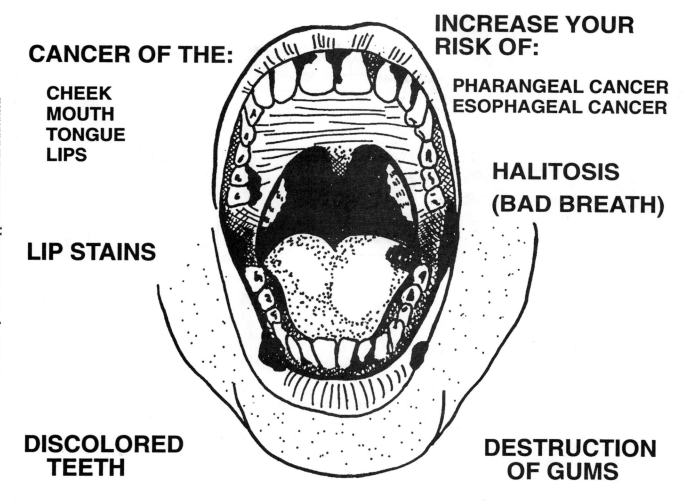

SOME CHEWING TOBACCOS CONTAIN MORE NICOTINE THAN CIGARETTES.

THE SURGEON GENERAL SAYS... (SA-29)

DIRECTIONS: Look in magazines that advertise cigarettes and list the various Surgeon General's warnings on the cigarette packs below. Make up your own warning in the space provided.

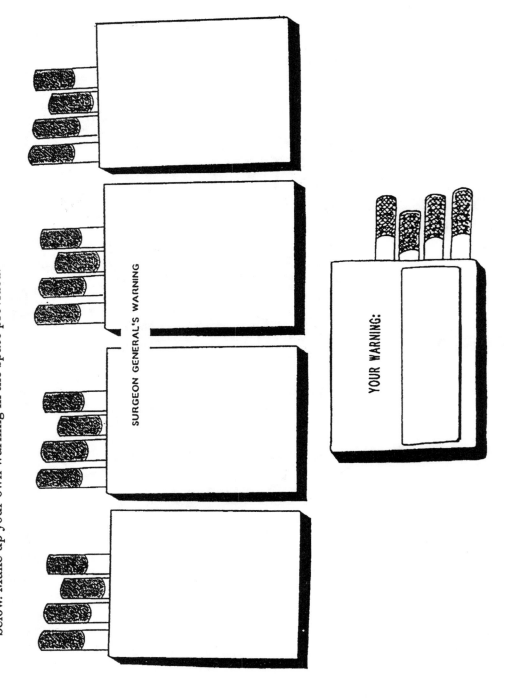

SURGEON GENERAL'S WARNING

YOUR WARNING:

GO FIGURE (SA-30)

DIRECTIONS: Find out the cost of a pack of cigarettes and figure out the answers to the problems below. Then, list all the items that you would like to have that are less than that dollar amount.

COST OF 1 PACK:

COST OF 1 PACK/DAY FOR 1 WEEK:

COST OF 1 PACK/DAY FOR 1 MONTH:

COST OF 1 PACK/DAY FOR 1 YEAR:

COST OF 1 PACK/DAY FOR 3 YEARS:

COST OF 1 PACK/DAY FOR 5 YEARS:

Items You Could Purchase Instead:

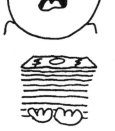

WOW....

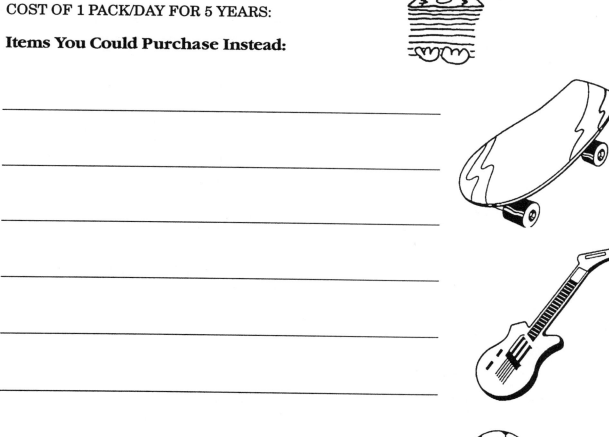

Name _____ Date _____

WHAT IS NICOTINE? (SA-31)

DIRECTIONS: Fill in the blanks with the correct word to make an accurate description of the drug nicotine. The pictures provide clues as to the word.

NICOTINE IS A _____ FOUND IN

THE _____ PLANT. IT IS

USED IN _____, _____,

_____, AND _____

TOBACCO. IF SMOKED, THE NICOTINE

ENTERS THE _____ AND THEN

THE BLOODSTREAM. IF _____,

IT MIXES WITH SALIVA AND GOES

INTO THE _____ AND SMALL

INTESTINES, THEN THE BLOODSTREAM.

IT IS ALSO ABSORBED THROUGH THE

LINING OF THE _____ INTO THE

BLOOD. NICOTINE IS A HIGHLY

ADDICTIVE, DANGEROUS DRUG.

DON'T SMOKE!

38

©1993 by The Center for Applied Research in Education

REASONS TO SMOKE

REASONS NOT TO SMOKE (SA-32)

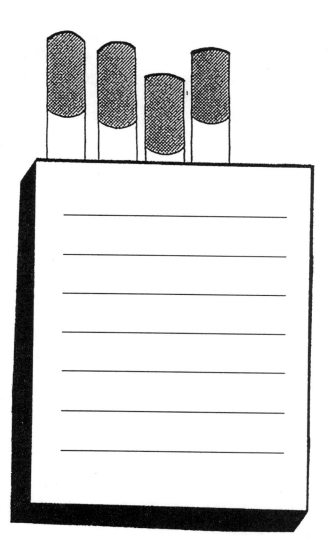

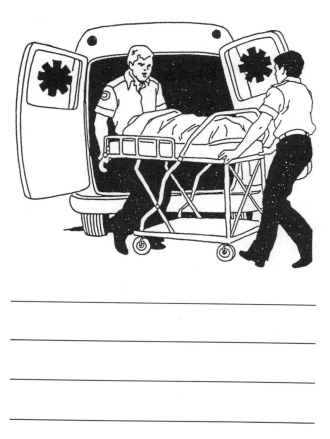

DIRECTIONS: On the lines provided, list all the reasons you can think of for smoking. Next list all the reasons you can think of for *not* smoking.

PACK IT IN!! (SA-33)

DIRECTIONS: Design your own brand of cigarettes highlighting the negative aspects of smoking. Cut out the pack when completed, mount it on construction paper, and display it with other packs.

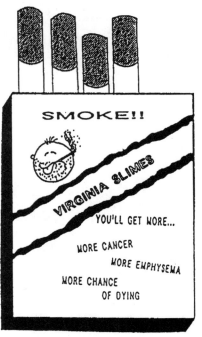

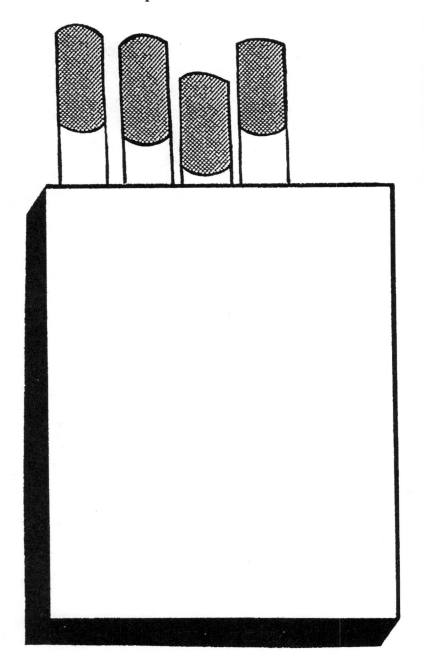

ACTIVITY 5 : WHAT IS...?
(Research on Lung Diseases)

Concept/ Description: Smoking cigarettes is a leading cause of death in the United States. Death most often occurs as a result of lung cancer, emphysema, or chronic bronchitis.

Objective: To have students research one of the three major lung diseases that cause death to many smokers and report their findings back to the class. To help students realize that these are preventable if a person chooses not to smoke.

Materials: What Is...? worksheet (SA-36)
Research books
Pamphlets from the American Cancer Society
Encyclopedias
Reference books
CD-ROM encyclopedias

Directions:
1. Assign each group, or individual, a particular disease and topic to research. For each of the three major diseases, assign a group to research the:
   a. causes of the disease;
   b. signs and symptoms;
   c. cures, or treatment;
   d. ways of preventing the disease of reducing your risks; or
   e. other facts or pertinent information.
2. Schedule a class visit to the library and ask the librarian to recommend materials on lung diseases, smoking, or both.
3. Give each student or group a What Is...? worksheet and have them research the topic assigned. Students should compile their information on the worksheet.
4. Use the diagram of the lungs to draw or label various characteristics of the disease, if desired.
5. Have the students report their findings back to the class.
6. Discuss why these preventable diseases are still killing people at an alarming rate. Ask students why they think smoking is accepted in our society when cigarettes kill more than 1,000 people each day.

Name _____ Date _____

WHAT IS... (SA-34)

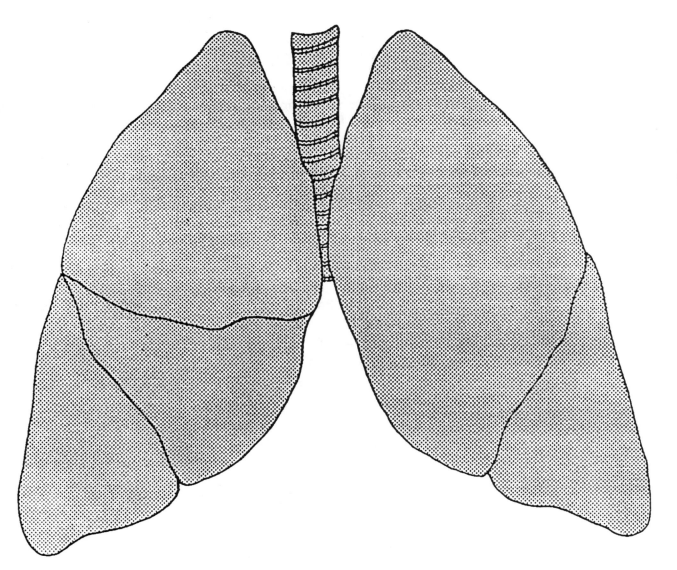

©1993 by The Center for Applied Research in Education

(Use the back of this sheet to write your report.)

CHRONIC BRONCHITIS? LUNG CANCER? EMPHYSEMA?

ACTIVITY 6 : LIGHT UP A MATCH!!
(Smoking Vocabulary Match-Game)

Concept/ Description: There are many difficult vocabulary words associated with smoking the respiratory system, and diseases.

Objective: To gain an understanding of the vocabulary associated with smoking by having students match the definition with the correct vocabulary word in a game format.

Materials: Match-Game Cards (SA-35–SA-39)
Scissors
Envelopes
Blank Match-Game Card Sheet (SA-40)

Directions:
1. Reproduce sets of the Match-Game Cards (forty cards per set on five sheets).
2. Cut out the cards (laminate first if you want a permanent set-up) and shuffle them.
3. Place a set of cards (forty cards) in an envelope.
4. Divide the class into groups of five or six and give each group its own set of cards in an envelope.
5. On the signal, have each group attempt to match the definition to its vocabulary word and place matched pairs on the floor.
6. Award points to the group that is finished first, second, third, etc. Do not award points until all the definitions are correct. Give points to all groups that finish correctly and additional points to the groups that finish the fastest.

Variations:
1. Give each member of the class a card. On the signal, see how quickly the students can find their partner.
2. Allow individuals to play a solitaire version of the game where they race against the clock. This works especially well at stations.

MATCH GAME CARDS (SA-35)

EMPHYSEMA	**AIR SACS IN THE LUNGS LOSE THEIR ELASTICITY**
NICOTINE	**ADDICTIVE SUBSTANCE IN TOBACCO**
CANCER	**ABNORMAL GROWTH OF CELLS**
CARBON MONOXIDE	**POISONOUS GAS PRODUCED BY TOBACCO SMOKE**

MATCH GAME CARDS (SA-36)

CHRONIC BRONCHITIS

EXCESSIVE SECRETIONS OF MUCUS IN THE BRONCHIAL TUBES

PEPTIC ULCER

AN OPEN SORE IN THE STOMACH LINING

SINUSITIS

SWELLING AND REDDENING OF THE SINUSES

CARDIOVASCULAR DISEASE

DISEASE OF THE HEART AND BLOOD VESSELS

LEUKOPLAKIA	**WHITE SPOTS ON THE INSIDE OF THE MOUTH THAT MAY BECOME CANCEROUS**
TAR	**DARK, STICKY SUBSTANCE IN TOBACCO THAT CAUSES CANCER**
BRONCHIOLES	**NARROW AIR TUBES IN THE LUNGS**
LUNGS	**ORGANS RESPONSIBLE FOR O_2 AND CO_2 EXCHANGE**

MATCH GAME CARDS (SA-38)

ALVEOLI

**AIR SACS
IN THE LUNGS**

CILIA

**TINY, HAIRLIKE
STRUCTURES THAT
FILTER OUT HARMFUL
SUBSTANCES IN THE
RESPIRATORY TRACT**

SNUFF

**FINELY GROUND
TOBACCO THAT
IS SNIFFED OR HELD
BETWEEN THE CHEEK
AND GUM**

ATHEROSCLEROSIS

**FATTY DEPOSITS
BLOCK THE ARTERIES**

HEMOGLOBIN	**SUBSTANCE IN RED BLOOD CELLS THAT CARRIES OXYGEN TO ALL CELLS**
CARCINOGEN	**CANCER-CAUSING AGENT**
ANOXIA	**DECREASE IN THE OXYGEN LEVEL IN THE BODY**
BENZOPYRENE	**CANCER-CAUSING CHEMICAL IN CIGARETTE SMOKE**

MAKE YOUR OWN CARDS (SA-40)

ACTIVITY 7: WHEN DID THAT HAPPEN?
(Smoking Time Line)

Concept/
Description: Since the early 1960s there have been many changes concerning cigarette smoking.

Objective: To have students determine the order of events described.

Materials: Smoking Time Line worksheet (SA-41)
Pen or pencil.

Directions:
1. Pass a Smoking Time Line worksheet to each student.
2. Have students research the events and then place them in the correct chronological order by writing the proper letter next to the corresponding date.
3. Discuss the impact of the various events, such as how banning cigarette advertising affected the tobacco industry.

Uhhh.....wasn't that in 200 B.C.?

SMOKING TIME LINE (SA-41)

DIRECTIONS: Write the letter of the event listed below next to the year that it occurred.

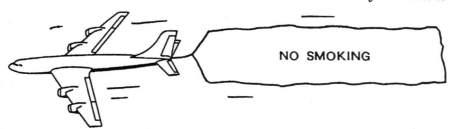

_____

_____ **1964**

_____

_____ **1965**

_____

_____ **1971**

_____

_____ **1972**

_____

_____ **1975**

_____

_____ **1983**

_____

_____ **1986**

_____

_____ **1988**

A. All U.S. airlines banned smoking on flights under two hours.

B. Minnesota passed the first state law requiring businesses, restaurants, and other institutions to establish no-smoking areas.

C. The Surgeon General declared that smoking causes lung cancer, respiratory diseases, and heart disease.

D. San Francisco became the first major city to limit smoking in the workplace.

E. The Surgeon General and the National Research Council linked secondhand smoke to lung cancer and respiratory disease in nonsmokers.

F. Warning labels are required on all cigarette packages.

G. The Surgeon General issued the first report indicating that secondhand smoke is dangerous to nonsmokers.

H. Cigarette makers withdrew advertisements from television and radio.

ACTIVITY 8: SAY IT LOUD AND CLEAR!
(Designing Anti-Smoking Buttons)

Concept/ Description: There are many reasons for not smoking.

Objective: To have students design an anti-smoking button based on information they have learned in class or through individual research.

Material: Button Design Sheet (SA-42)
Markers, colored pencils, crayons
Scissors
Access to a laminating machine (optional)
Tape

Directions:
1. Give each student a Button Design Sheet.
2. Have students design a button using the illustrations given, or they can design their own.
3. Each button should be easily readable and clear.
4. If available, laminate the buttons for display in the classroom or to wear (use a rolled piece of tape).

Variations:
1. Vote for the best design and distribute them to the faculty or students.
2. Enlarge the design and have students color them in and display throughout the school.
3. Purchase a button making machine and make actual buttons. (These are available in many art supply or student council fundraising catalogues).

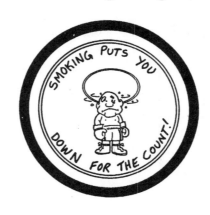

Name _____   Date _____

BUTTON DESIGN SHEET (SA-42)

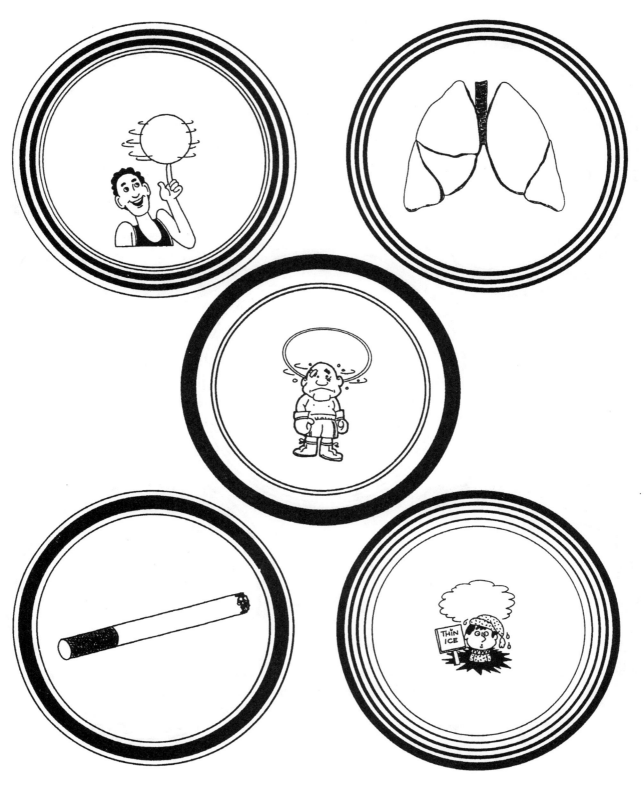

Name _____ Date _____

BUTTON DESIGN SHEET (SA-43)

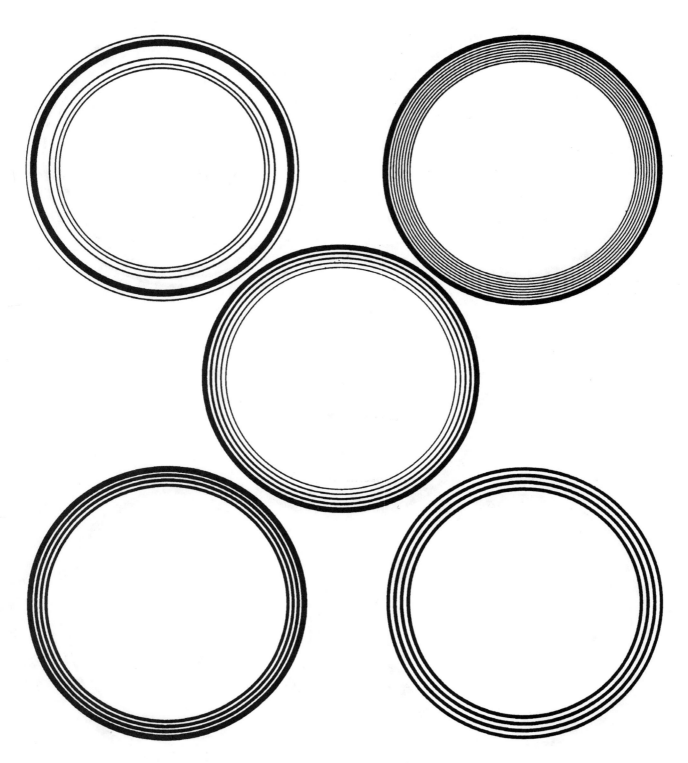

TOPICS FOR DISCUSSION (SA-44)

SMOKING

DIRECTIONS: Discuss these topics with your group and be prepared to report your group's feelings back to the class.

1. Should smoking be banned from all public places?

2. Should tobacco companies be allowed to sponsor sporting events? (Example: Virginia Slims Tennis Tounament)

3. Should our government continue to subsidize tobacco farmers?

4. Should people who develop lung cancer or other fatal diseases from smoking be allowed to sue the tobacco companies?

5. Should smoking sections be permitted on airlines?

6. Should all tobacco advertising be banned? (billboards, magazines, sporting events, etc.)

7. Should people be required to pay higher taxes on cigarettes than they already pay? Should the money go to cancer research?

8. Should a company be allowed to fire an employee who smokes? Under what circumstances, if any?

9. Do smokers have rights? What are they?

10. Do nonsmokers have rights? What are they?

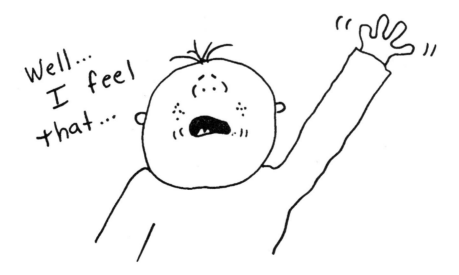

DRUGS

- **Understanding Methods and Types of Drugs**

- **Information Please! (Profiles of Drugs)**

- **Types of Drug Abuse**

- **Checking Comprehension: Drug Abuse**

Name _____   **Date** _____

HOW DRUGS ENTER THE BLOODSTREAM (SA-45)

DIRECTIONS: Using the words listed below, fill in the blanks to explain how drugs enter the bloodstream.

alveoli	bloodstream	muscle
stomach	capillaries	nasal
under	vein	vessels

1. **TAKEN BY MOUTH**

   The drug passes through the walls of the _____ and then into the small

   intestine to be absorbed into the _____ .

2. **INHALED**

   The drug enters the bloodstream by way of the rich supply of blood _____ in

   the _____ passages.

3. **SMOKED**

   The drug passes from the _____ (sacs) in the lungs into the _____
   and the bloodstream.

4. **APPLIED TO THE SKIN**

   The drug is applied to the skin, passes through the pores and into the tiny capillaries and
   the bloodstream.

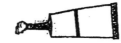

5. **INJECTED**

   a. **Skin Popping**—the drug is injected _____ the skin.

   b. **Intramuscular Injection**—the drug is injected deep into a _____ .

   c. **Mainlining**—the drug is injected directly into a _____ .

WHY PEOPLE ABUSE DRUGS (SA-46)

DIRECTIONS: Fill in the missing letters to give reasons why some people abuse drugs.

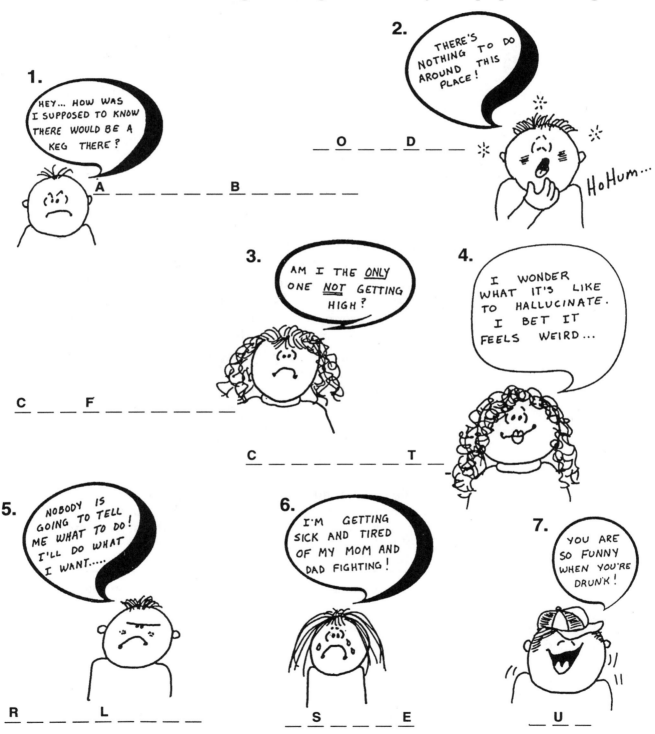

ACTIVITY 9: CATEGORIES
(Understanding Drug Types)

Concept/
Description: Different substances produce different effects on the body systems.

Objectives: To have students identify which types of drugs produce certain reactions in a game format.

Materials: Index Cards
Tape
Substance Sheet (SA-47)
Blackboard, chalk

Directions:
1. Write the words listed on the Substance Sheet onto the index cards (one substance per card).
2. Diagram the blackboard as shown in Figure 1.
3. Divide the class into groups of three or four students and give each group some of the cards.
4. Have each group, in turn, tape a card to the blackboard under the category to which they think it belongs.
5. Award one point for each correct answer. If a substance is placed on the board in the wrong category, the next group up may elect to correct the answer for one point and then put their card up for an additional point. If the group that corrects the answer is also wrong, they lose their turn and may not put up a card until the next round.
6. The team with the most points is declared the winner.

Variation:
1. Use the street names of the various drugs and have students place them under the correct headings. You may wish to let students research the drugs to find out the street names. (See SA-48 as a teacher reference.)

DEPRESSANTS	STIMULANTS	HALLUCINOGENS	NARCOTICS	INHALANTS	MARIJUANA

Figure 1.

SUBSTANCE SHEET (SA-47)

NARCOTICS

codeine
Demerol
Dilaudid
heroin
methadone
morphine
opium
Percodan
Talwin
Darvon
paregoric

STIMULANTS

Benzedrine
Dexedrine
Methadrine
cocaine
caffeine
nicotine
crack

DEPRESSANTS

wine
beer
hard liquor
Quaaludes
Tuinal
Seconal
Amytal
Nembutal
Phenobarbital
Sopor
Librium
Valium
Thorazine

HALLUCINOGENS

LSD
mescaline
peyote
psilocybin
PCP
MDA

INHALANTS

amyl nitrite
butyl nitrite
nitrous oxide
glue
gasoline
cleaning fluid
nail polish remover
aerosol spray
laquer
liquid correction fluid
spot remover

MARIJUANA

hashish
THC
Thai stick
sinsemilla

STREET NAMES SHEET (SA-48)

NARCOTICS

schoolboy
demies
little D
smack
junk
downtown
meth
dollies
M
Miss Emma
morph
blue velvet
black stuff
perkies
Ts
scag
horse
dope

STIMULANTS

bennies
black beauties
co-pilots
dexies
speed
meth
crank
uppers
coke
snow
blow
nose candy
toot
uptown
whites
ups
Christmas trees
hearts

DEPRESSANTS

blues
downers
yellow jackets
yellows
phennies
purple hearts
reds
F-40s
rainbows
D
downers
ludes
714s
Qs
sopors
red devils
redbirds
blue heaven
tooeys
barbs
downs
booze

HALLUCINOGENS

acid
purple haze
blue cheer
angel dust
super grass
killer weed
scramblers
blotter
buttons
cubes
shrooms
mesc
cactus
magic mushrooms
window panes
the love drug

INHALANTS

popper
bolt
locker room
rush
ames
laughing gas

MARIJUANA

pot
grass
weed
joints
jays
sticks
Mary Jane
reefer
roach
hash
kif
herb
ganja
Acapulco gold
Panama red
Columbian
Maui wowee

MARIJUANA PRE-TEST (SA-49)

DIRECTIONS: Place a *T* for True or an *F* for False in the blank to the left.

_____ 1. Marijuana can be eaten or smoked.

_____ 2. Though THC is the main ingredient in pot, when smoked pot produces over 2,000 chemicals.

_____ 3. THC will remain in the body for up to 12 hours.

_____ 4. Marijuana smoke contains more cancer-causing chemicals than cigarette smoke.

_____ 5. Marijuana is stored in the fatty tissue surrounding the reproductive organs, the lungs, and the brain.

_____ 6. The marijuana sold today is a lot weaker than that sold in the 1960s.

_____ 7. Marijuana used in small amounts (one joint or less) is legal.

_____ 8. Marijuana could lead to the use of other drugs.

_____ 9. The more pot you smoke, the less you need to get high.

_____10. Marijuana is legal in some states in the U.S.

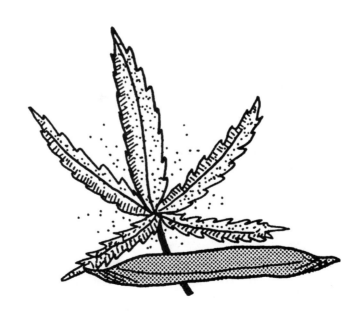

Name _____   **Date** _____

REASONS TO USE DRUGS

REASONS NOT TO USE DRUGS (SA-50)

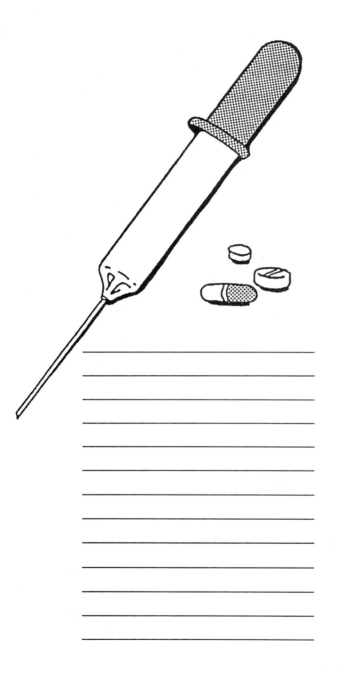

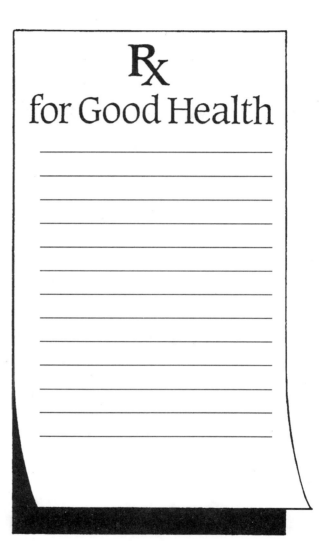

DIRECTIONS: On the lines provided, list all the reasons you can think of for using illegal drugs. Next list all the reasons you can think of for *not* using drugs.

ACTIVITY 10: WHAT IS CAFFEINE? WHERE IS IT FOUND?
(Product Survey)

Concept/ Description: Caffeine is a white, odorless, bitter substance that occurs naturally. It is a stimulant found in many products we use. Small amounts of caffeine increase the blood circulation, and large amounts can cause stomach upsets, headaches, heart palpitations, nervousness, and loss of sleep. Though caffeine use hasn't been conclusively linked to major heath problems, many doctors advise pregnant women to reduce their intake of the substance.

Objective: To have students see first-hand which products contain caffeine.

Materials: Caffeine Product Survey (SA-51)

Directions:
1. Have individuals or groups of students complete the Caffeine Product Survey at local food stores.
2. Explain that when surveying soft drinks the students should look for 12-ounce cans. Coffee and cocoa should be based on 8-ounce cups, and tea based on 5-ounce cups. (You may vary this if you wish.)
3. When comparing chocolate, look for 1-ounce bars.
4. Under each picture on the survey sheet, students should list product names in that category that contain caffeine. List the number of milligrams of caffeine next to the product name.

   EXAMPLE: "Mountain Dew, 50 mg."
5. If the amount of caffeine isn't listed clearly, students should call the toll-free number listed on the product and request the information.
6. After the surveys are completed, compile a list of the results and discuss.

Coffee?

I've had enough coffee, thank you!

Name _____   Date _____

CAFFEINE PRODUCT SURVEY (SA-51)

DIRECTIONS: Place the brand names of products containing caffeine under the corresponding headings. Next to each brand name list the number of milligrams of caffeine.

COFFEE

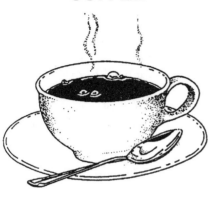

SOFT DRINKS

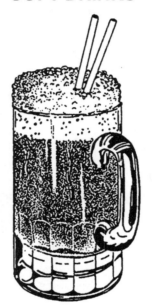

TEA

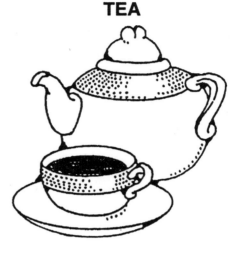

PAIN RELIEVERS

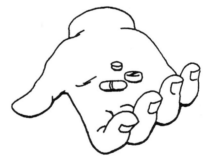

CHOCOLATE

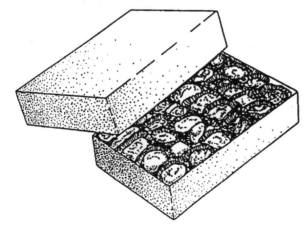

COCOA

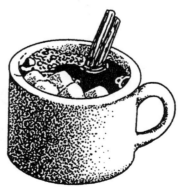

INFORMATION PLEASE!

The following reproducibles may be used by the teacher as reference materials or may be given to students for individual research or to assist in note taking during a lecture.

Another way to use the sheets is to have groups research the assigned topics, write their information on the sheets, and display the sheets in your classroom.

The answers to the sheets are located in the answer key at the back of the book.

SA-52: Marijuana

SA-53: Narcotics

SA-54: Inhalants

SA-55: Cocaine

SA-56: Hallucinogens

SA-57: Depressants

SA-58: Stimulants

SA-59: Anabolic Steroids

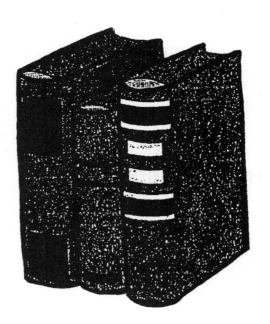

MARIJUANA (SA-52)

DRUGS:

DESCRIPTION:

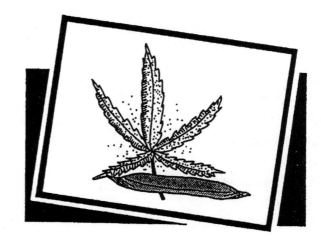

SLANG NAMES:

HOW IT ENTERS THE BODY:

EFFECTS:

MEDICAL USE:

NARCOTICS (SA-53)

DRUGS:

DESCRIPTION:

SLANG NAMES:

HOW IT ENTERS THE BODY:

EFFECTS:

MEDICAL USE:

INHALANTS (SA-54)

DRUGS:

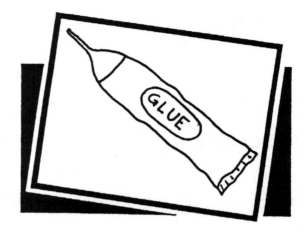

DESCRIPTION:

SLANG NAMES:

HOW IT ENTERS THE BODY:

EFFECTS:

MEDICAL USE:

©1993 by The Center for Applied Research in Education

COCAINE (SA-55)

DRUGS:

DESCRIPTION:

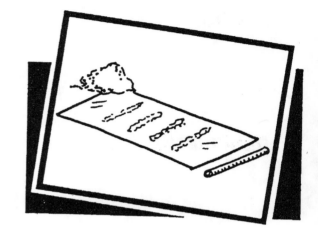

SLANG NAMES:

HOW IT ENTERS THE BODY:

EFFECTS:

MEDICAL USE:

HALLUCINOGENS (SA-56)

DRUGS:

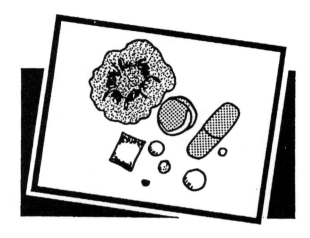

DESCRIPTION:

SLANG NAMES:

HOW IT ENTERS THE BODY:

EFFECTS:

MEDICAL USE:

DEPRESSANTS (SA-57)

DRUGS:

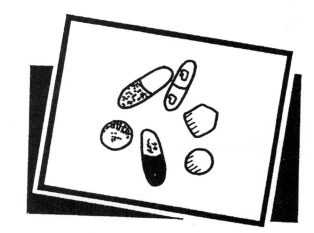

DESCRIPTION:

SLANG NAMES:

HOW IT ENTERS THE BODY:

EFFECTS:

MEDICAL USE:

STIMULANTS (SA-58)

DRUGS:

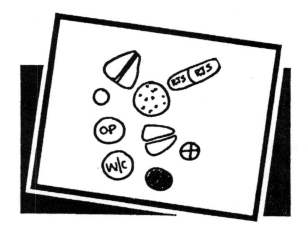

DESCRIPTION:

SLANG NAMES:

HOW IT ENTERS THE BODY:

EFFECTS:

MEDICAL USE:

ANABOLIC STEROIDS (SA-59)

DRUGS:

DESCRIPTION:

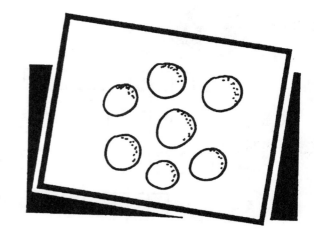

SLANG NAMES:

HOW IT ENTERS THE BODY:

EFFECTS:

MEDICAL USE:

DRUG VOCABULARY CROSSWORD (SA-60)

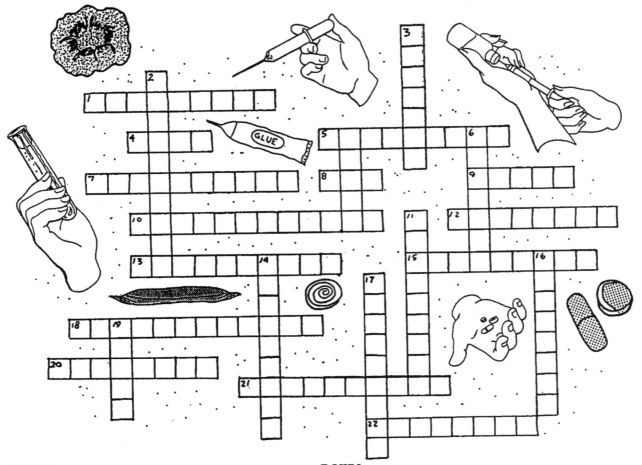

ACROSS

1. Two drugs combine to produce effects much greater than if each was used alone.
4. Any substance that chemically affects the mind or body.
5. Drugs that are derived from the opium poppy.
7. Hallucinations that occur days, weeks, and months after the drug has been used.
8. A reason for using drugs.
9. A potent form of cocaine sold in ready-to-smoke rocks.
10. Drug that causes the mind to see or imagine things that aren't real.
12. An addictive stimulant found in tobacco.
13. Drugs that speed up body systems.
15. Going against authority; a reason to use drugs.
18. Instructions by a doctor to a pharmacist.
20. Feeling of lightheadedness or being "high."
21. Removal of a drug from the body systems. This often causes physical or psychological distress.
22. A stimulant found in tea, cola, chocolate, and coffee.

DOWN

2. A type of drug that slows down body systems.
3. The most abused substance in the United States.
6. An expensive white powder that comes from the leaves of the coca bush.
11. A drug that is smoked or eaten and is also called pot, weed, and grass.
14. Needing a drug in order to survive.
16. Substance that is sniffed in order to get "high" from the fumes.
17. Needing more and more of a drug to feel its effects.
19. The type of alcohol used in beverages.

I'M BORED!!
(SA-61)

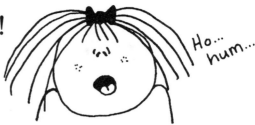

Ho... hum...

DIRECTIONS: In the blocks shown below, draw and label the eight activities that you enjoy doing most. Put an asterisk (*) next to your favorite. Compare your paper with a partner's and compile a list of activities to do besides drugs.

W H A T   T O   D O   B E S I D E S   D R U G S

ACTIVITY 11: PORTRAIT OF A DRUG ADDICT
(Types of Drug Abuse)

Concept/ Description: There are many types of drug abusers and knowing the "stages" can help in understanding the dangers.

Objective: To have students see the profound changes from experimentation to addiction.

Materials: Types of Drug Abuse worksheets (SA-62 and SA-63)
Types of Drug Abuse Transparencies (SA-64 to SA-67)
Overhead projector

Directions:
1. Before class begins, have the Types of Drug Abuse transparencies (SA-64 to SA-67) transferred onto transparency film using a thermal copy machine, or trace them onto acetate.
2. Pass out a Types of Drug Abuse (SA-62-63) worksheet to each student.
3. Have students fill in the worksheet with the information placed on the overhead projector.
4. Explain each type of abuse as you proceed.
5. Discuss whether a person who is using would believe that they were in danger. Why or why not?
6. Discuss whether every user could become an addict. Why or why not?
7. What excuses might a user give for using?

Name _____ **Date** _____

TYPES OF DRUG ABUSE (SA-62)

THE EXPERIMENTER

1. _____ is a motivator.

2. The user is learning about the _____ _____ brought on by the drug.

3. The user is learning to _____ / _____ the drug and its effects.

4. Getting _____ is a new feeling not in the normal range of emotions.

5. The user can still _____ to people.

REGULAR USER

1. The decision to _____ has been made.

2. The user now seeks the _____ .

3. There is increased _____ and _____ in the use of the drug.

4. The _____ group that the person hangs out with uses.

5. Getting "high" is more _____ now.

6. _____ develops.

7. The person becomes _____.

8. The user has some problems _____ to others.

TYPES OF DRUG ABUSE (*continued*) (SA-63)

PREOCCUPIED USER

1. The user is _____ more about drugs.

2. The user wants to be "high" _____ .

3. _____ start to occur.

4. Relationships are _____.

5. The person clearly wants to _____ _____ _____.

6. The person uses when _____, which is very dangerous.

7. The user still thinks he or she has _____.

THE ADDICT

1. The addict can _____ _____ get "high."

2. The user must take the drug to _____.

3. There is no _____ : you must use.

4. The person relates to _____ ,

   not to _____.

5. The addict will use _____ _____.

6. The behavior is both obnoxious and _____.

7. _____ are the user's life.

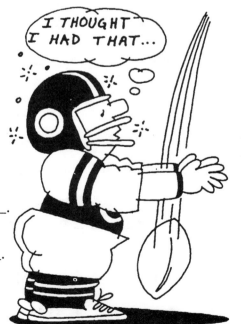

TYPES OF DRUG ABUSE (SA-64)

THE EXPERIMENTER

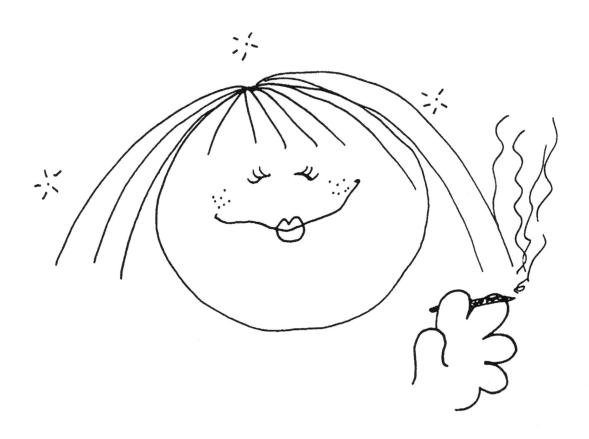

CURIOSITY IS A MOTIVATOR
LEARNING ABOUT THE MOOD SWINGS
LEARNING TO TRUST/MISTRUST THE DRUG
"HIGH" IS A NEW FEELING
CAN STILL RELATE TO PEOPLE

TYPES OF DRUG ABUSE (SA-65)

REGULAR USER

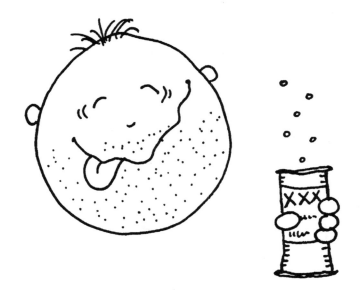

**THE DECISION TO USE HAS BEEN MADE
SEEKS THE "HIGH"
COMFORT AND CONFIDENCE IN USING
PEER GROUP USES
GETTING "HIGH" IS MORE IMPORTANT
TOLERANCE DEVELOPS
COCKY
HAS SOME PROBLEMS RELATING**

PREOCCUPIED USER

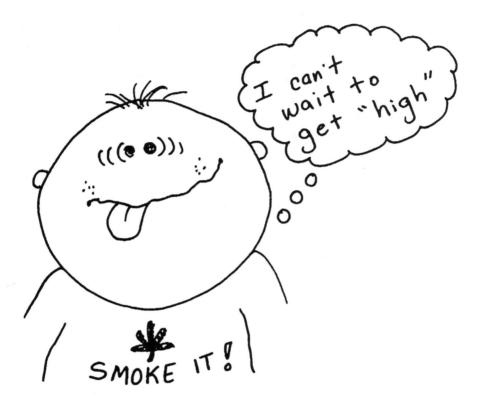

THINKING MORE ABOUT DRUGS
WANTS TO BE "HIGH" OFTEN
BLACKOUTS START
RELATIONSHIPS ARE DIFFICULT
CLEARLY WANTS TO USE THE DRUG
USES WHEN ALONE
STILL THINKS IS IN CONTROL

TYPES OF DRUG ABUSE (SA-67)

THE ADDICT

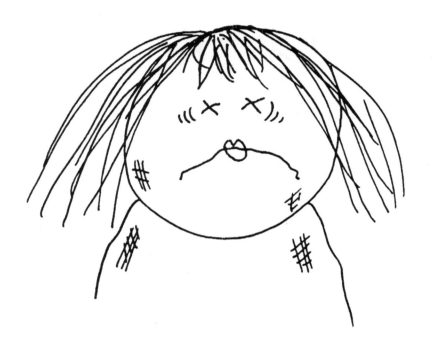

**CAN NO LONGER GET "HIGH"
MUST TAKE DRUG TO SURVIVE
NO CHOICE: MUST USE
RELATES TO DRUGS, NOT PEOPLE
WILL USE ANY TIME
OBNOXIOUS, INTIMIDATING
DRUGS ARE YOUR LIFE**

VOCAB-A-MANIA (SA-68)

DIRECTIONS: Match the word with its definition and place the correct letter in the blank to the left.

_____ 1. emphysema
_____ 2. caffeine
_____ 3. blackout
_____ 4. anabolic steroids
_____ 5. tolerance
_____ 6. reverse tolerance
_____ 7. seizure
_____ 8. judgment
_____ 9. HGH
_____ 10. hallucination
_____ 11. euphoria
_____ 12. ethyl
_____ 13. cirrhosis
_____ 14. paranoia
_____ 15. BAC
_____ 16. PCP
_____ 17. tar
_____ 18. nicotine
_____ 19. carbon monoxide
_____ 20. ice
_____ 21. withdrawal
_____ 22. addiction

a. compulsive use of a drug which causes physical and psychological dependence
b. synthetic hormones used by some athletes to increase muscle mass
c. a highly addictive, smokable form of "speed"
d. a disease of the lungs often caused by smoking
e. type of alcohol in alcoholic beverages
f. the ingredient in tobacco that causes addiction
g. phencyclidine, "angel dust," a potent hallucinogen
h. a liver disease that is often the result of drinking heavily for many years
i. a poisonous gas found in cigarette smoke
j. the stimulant found in coffee, tea, chocolate, and colas
k. excessive and irrational distrust of others sometimes brought on by certain types of drugs
l. needing more and more of a substance to feel its effects
m. unpleasant physical and psychological symptoms brought on by discontinuing the use of a drug
n. the ingredient in tobacco that causes cancer
o. an abnormal, violent contraction of muscles, or a convulsion sometimes due to drug use
p. the amount of alcohol in the bloodstream
q. loss of memory without passing out
r. elation or feeling of extreme well-being
s. sensory distortion
t. human growth hormone
u. the ability to form an opinion or make an evaluation
v. needing less of a drug to feel "high"

Name _____ **Date** _____

A TALE OF WOE (SA-69)

DIRECTIONS: Correct the story below by writing the correct word or words above the underlined word.

Fast Eddie, an internationally known drug dealer, had a rough day out on the street. The wanted criminal had a kilo of heroin stolen from his car—that's <u>5.2</u> pounds of the <u>stimulant</u> that comes from the <u>coca bush</u>! When Fast Eddie went to the police, they were far from sympathetic, in fact they arrested him on the spot. It seems they discovered crack in his pocket. Crack is a smokable form of <u>glue</u>. Fast Eddie also had too much to drink. The police gave him a breathalyzer test which measures the amount of <u>nicotine</u> in the <u>urine</u> and found his BAC to be .20 percent, which is legally intoxicated.

Fast Eddie was sent to jail, but that didn't stop him. He sat down and lit up a joint, which is a cigarette containing <u>opium</u>. The police officer in charge stopped him immediately. She suggested that Fast Eddie join a support group such as NA which stands for <u>Nutrition</u> Anonymous. Eddie promised to do that as soon as he got out of jail.

Two years later Fast Eddie was released and, as promised, joined NA and is now recovering. In fact, Eddie hasn't touched alcohol or other drugs at all. He said the hardest part of recovery was <u>tolerance</u>, which is when the drug is removed from the body systems. Eddie has a long road ahead of him, but Eddie is doing much better and is happy to be drug and alcohol free.

Here's a little help...

NARCOTICS
withdrawal
alcohol
2.2
opium poppy
depressant
3.5
marijuana
cocaine
synergism
bloodstream
narcotic
hallucinogen

GENERAL ACTIVITIES

- **Advertising that Promotes Drugs**

- **How Drugs Affect the Fetus**

- **Legal Consequences of Drug Use**

- **A Letter to a Friend**

- **Forming Opinions**

- **Understanding Denial**

- **Seeking Help**

ACTIVITY 12: CAVEAT EMPTOR
(Let the Buyer Beware)

Concept/ Description: If we understand the types of advertising ploys manufacturers use, we may be less likely to believe everything we see or hear.

Objective: To have the students be able to identify various advertising gimmicks used to promote cigarettes and alcohol.

Materials: Magazines that have cigarette and alcohol ads.
Ad Questionnaire (SA-70)
Advertising Techniques Sheet (SA-71)

Directions:
1. Pass out an Ad Questionnaire and an Advertising Techniques Sheet to each student.
2. Have students work in groups and give each group a pile of magazines.
3. Each group is to tear out the ads on cigarettes and alcohol.
4. Have the students fill out the Ad Questionnaire based on any cigarette or alcohol ad.
5. Discuss the ads and the types of techniques the advertisers seem to use the most for each type of product. Is beer advertised the same way that liquor is advertised? What type of advertising do cigarette manufacturers often employ?

Variation: Do the same activity, but instead of using magazine ads, videotape TV ads and have students discuss and evaluate each ad after it is shown. Have students refer to the Advertising Techniques Sheet during the discussion.

I LIKE THE AIR JORDAN COMMERCIALS!

Name _____ **Date** _____

AD QUESTIONNAIRE (SA-70)

1. What TV commercial is your favorite? Briefly describe.

2. Why?

3. Refer to the Advertising Techniques Sheet and list the technique that your favorite ad uses:

Choose an alcohol or cigarette ad from a magazine and answer the following questions:

1. What product is being advertised?

2. Does the ad give any factual information about the product? If so, what?

3. Are there people present in the ad? If so, what are they doing?

4. To whom do you think this ad is geared? (Adults? Men? Women? Teenagers?)

5. What, according to the ad, will this product supposedly do for you?

6. What advertising techniques are being used?

7. Do you like the ad? Why or why not?

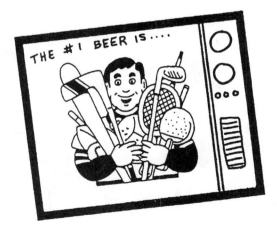

ADVERTISING TECHNIQUES (SA-71)

1. **Testimonial.** An authoritative person such as a doctor or athlete may testify that they use the product; therefore, you should too. The ad may have nothing at all to do with the product's quality.

2. **Sense Appeal.** Pictures or sounds are used to appeal to the senses. For example, a hamburger sizzles on a hot grill or an ice cold beer is poured into a frosty mug.

3. **Transfer.** A sexy, well-dressed, or popular looking person sells the product. The buyer imagines that they will gain those attributes if they use the product.

4. **Bandwagon.** The ad suggests that "everyone" uses the product and that the buyer better go along with it or they'll be left out.

5. **Plainfolks.** An average, down-home, back-to-basics person advertises the product so that the average buyer identifies with the product.

6. **Humor.** People tend to remember commercials that make them laugh and therefore associate a positive feeling with the product.

7. **Statistics.** People tend to be impressed by statistics. Many ads leave out important details of the statistics, however. For example: Who conducted a particular study? Who was polled? Where was the study done?

8. **Cardstacking.** Advertisers give a one-sided view of their product, leaving out the bad or negative aspects and concentrating only on the good.

9. **Public Good.** Ads claim their product is in the best interest of the consumer, society, or the world; or they associate it with "good" things such as freedom, recycling, saving the rainforests, baby seals, etc.

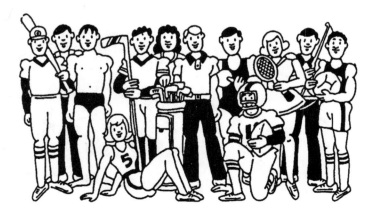

OH BABY! 1 (SA-72)

DIRECTIONS: Place the words given below into the story to explain how drugs can affect the fetus.

COCAINE

seizures	premature	SIDS	kidneys
miscarriages	stillbirths	placenta	retards
	withdrawal	shock	

The use of cocaine by women in the early months of pregnancy can cause _____

or _____ . In later months, it may cause _____ delivery.

Cocaine _____ fetal growth and head size, and can cause malformed

_____ and genitals. Cocaine increases the risk of _____ , Sudden

Infant Death Syndrome. It may cause premature separation of the _____ from the

uterus resulting in heavy bleeding and _____ . Many cocaine babies are born going

through _____ and suffering _____ .

MARIJUANA

| length | fat | tremors | longer |
| THC | weight | visual | |

The use of marijuana during pregnancy can result in low birth _____ and

_____ . _____ , the active ingredient in marijuana, remains in the fetal

brain _____ than in the mother's brain because the fetus's brain has a higher

_____ content. Marijuana use can cause the baby to have _____ at

birth, seizures, and _____ problems.

OH BABY! 2 (SA-73)

ALCOHOL

facial	sex organs	Fetal Alcohol Syndrome
hyperactivity	no safe level	sleep
retardation	heart	below-normal

Alcohol use can cause _____ (FAS), which is characterized by retarded fetal growth and infants who are born with _____ weight and size. FAS includes _____ deformity: small head, narrow eyes, flat nose, thin upper lip. Alcohol can also cause defects and deformity of the _____ , kidneys, muscles, joints, and _____ . It can cause mental _____ , learning disorders, _____ , lack of coordination, and _____ disturbances. There is _____ of use during pregnancy.

TOBACCO

six	heart	bloodstream	oxygen
increases	chemicals	lung	death
	smoke	most	

Tobacco _____ contains thousands of different _____ that cross the placenta and enter the fetus's _____ . As a result, the amount of _____ to the fetus is reduced and the risk of miscarriage increases. The chance of infant _____ in the first year also _____ . Other negative effects include low birth weight, delivery problems, and a higher chance of infant _____ and _____ disease. Tobacco is the _____ damaging in the last _____ months of pregnancy.

ACTIVITY 13: IT'S THE LAW!
(Legal Consequences of Drug Use)

Concept/ Description: There are legal as well as physical consequences you must face if you choose to use drugs.

Objective: To understand the consequences of illegal drug use.

Materials: None

Directions:
1. Invite a local district attorney or law enforcement official to speak to your class about the penalties for underage drinking, drug use, etc.

2. Ask the speaker to specifically address these issues:

   - drugs or drinking and driving
   - selling drugs
   - underage drinking
   - possession of drugs and alcohol
   - using a fake ID
   - making and selling fake IDs
   - purchasing tobacco or alcohol
   - protection from drunk drivers

3. Allow students to come up with their own questions and topics to discuss.

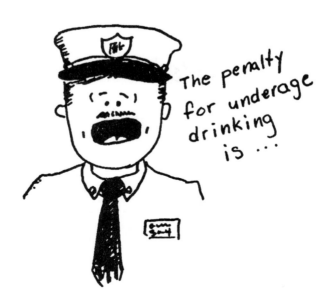

ACTIVITY 14: DEAR JOHN . . .
(A Letter to a Friend)

Concept/
Description: Helping a friend can sometimes help you to see problems more clearly.

Objective: Students will write a letter to a fictional friend in a rehab to offer support.

Materials: Paper
Pens or pencils
List of Fictional Friends (see SA-74)

Directions: 1. Pass out or read the Fictional Friends handout and ask students to choose one person on the list.
2. Ask the students to write a letter to that person offering support, advice, or suggestions.
3. Ask volunteers to read the letter to the class.
4. Discuss the problems the Fictional Friends may face when they leave rehab.

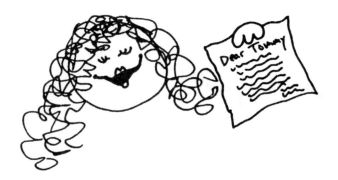

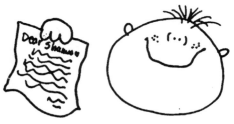

FICTIONAL FRIENDS (SA-74)

1. **John Williams.** John is 16 and has always been in trouble at school. He is fun to be around, but has become very angry lately. Everyone at school knows he gets "high" before school. His mom drinks all the time and his dad left years ago. John placed himself in rehab last week.

2. **Shannon Smith.** Shannon was dating a popular football player at school who is two years older than she is. She began to drink because her boyfriend did, but now she can't seem to stop. Her boyfriend dumped her last month. Shannon's parents noticed that Shannon was stealing liquor from the liquor cabinet, and placed her in rehab.

3. **Bill Johnson.** Bill is a high school senior who is the life of the party. He is always drunk at parties and makes the whole crowd laugh. Last week he drove his car off the road and seriously injured some children playing. He is receiving a mandatory drug and alcohol evaluation, and it has been recommended that Bill remain in rehab.

4. **Linda Jones.** Linda is 13 years old, but hangs out with her 16-year-old brother's friends. She started getting high on a dare, but then decided that drugs made her confident and it was no longer difficult to talk to people. Linda was caught passing out "ludes" to her friends at school. She was sent to rehab.

5. **Tommy McNally.** Tommy always tries to be the drunkest or higher than anyone else, and usually is. Tommy is a very good athlete, but would rather get "loaded" than go to practice every day. Tommy got involved with cocaine and quickly developed an addiction. Tommy asked some friends for help and now he's in rehab. He's having a difficult time but really wants to stop using drugs.

ACTIVITY 15: SAVE THE BEST FOR LAST
(Rank Ordering)

Concept/Description: Individuals form opinions based on many factors. Some of those factors are environment, parents, and friends. This activity generates discussion based on those varied opinions.

Objective: Students will rank individuals described from most negative traits to least negative traits based on their personal opinions.

Materials: Save the Best for Last worksheets (SA-75 and SA-76).
Pens or pencils

Directions:
1. Give each student a Save the Best for Last worksheet.
2. Have the students rank (from 1 to 10) the people described.
3. After all students have finished, list the rankings on the board.

   • Which person generated the most negative votes (1, 2, or 3)?
   • Which person was least offensive to your class?

4. Discuss why the students chose the people they did.
5. Ask them to speculate on how past experience may influence someone's opinion. Ask for examples.

Variation: Have students give a Save the Best for Last worksheet to a parent to fill out. Compare student and parent responses. Why is there a difference in responses? Discuss.

SAVE THE BEST FOR LAST (SA-75)

DIRECTIONS: Rank the people listed below based on how strongly you feel about the negative traits described. Number 1 is the person you feel has the *most* negative traits and number 10 has the *fewest* negative traits.

PERSON	DESCRIPTION	RANK
Mrs. Smith, guidance counselor	A student comes into Mrs. Smith's office for advice about her drinking and Mrs. Smith tells the student's parents.	_____
Hypocrite Mom	Mom uses diet pills and tranquilizers and chain smokes. She grounds her son for trying booze.	_____
Party Dude	Rick comes to every school dance drunk and never gets caught.	_____
Pot Head Brother	A 16-year-old turns his 11-year-old brother on to pot.	_____
Officer McNally	A policeman knows of an 8th grade drinking party but doesn't do anything about it.	_____

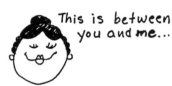

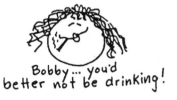

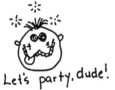

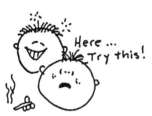

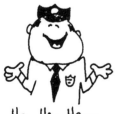

SAVE THE BEST FOR LAST *(continued)* (SA-76)

Coach Bubba

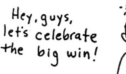

A high school football coach drinks with his team to celebrate a big win.

_____

Drunk Driver

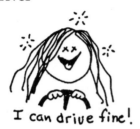

An 18-year-old girl has been drinking heavily, but insists on driving everyone home.

_____

Burn Out

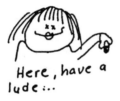

A person at school passes out a bunch of her mom's tranquilizers to her friends.

_____

Drunk Dad

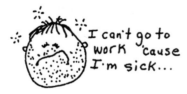

A father cannot hold down a job because he's always drunk, and now his family may lose their house.

_____

Ms. Brown

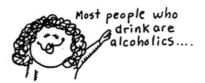

A teacher at school tells lies about drugs so that her students will be afraid to try them.

_____

ACTIVITY 16: SUBSTANCE ABUSE PREVENTION GAME

Concept/Description: Using a game to review material helps students reinforce their learning.

Objective: To score points by coming up with questions to fit given answers.

Materials: Substance Abuse Prevention Game sheet (SA-77)
Pens or pencils
Substance Abuse Answer Key (SA-78)

Directions:
1. Give individuals, or groups of two or three, a Substance Abuse Prevention Game sheet.
2. Students fill in the blocks with the correct questions. (You may wish to allow the use of notes.)
3. If you do not wish to make this a competitive game, simply collect the papers and add up the points.
4. To make the game competitive, you may do the following:
   a. Set a time limit by putting times on the board with bonus point values. For example, if the paper is finished between 2:00 and 2:15, and all answers are correct, the group (or person) gets 10 bonus points; if done between 2:15 and 2:30, the group gets 8 points, etc.

      NOTE: Be sure to have the answer key readily available.
   b. Rather than a time limit, give the first paper turned in with all answers correct 10 bonus points; second paper in gets 8 points, etc.

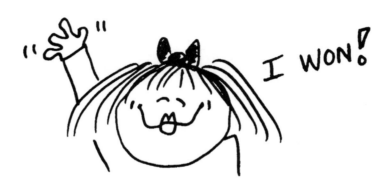

Name _____   Date _____

SUBSTANCE ABUSE PREVENTION GAME (SA-77)

		DRUGS	ALCOHOL	TOBACCO	DISEASES	GENERAL
10 pts.	?					
	A	Category of drugs that come from the opium poppy.	Double the percentage of alcohol in a beverage.	Stimulant found in tobacco.	Tiny hairlike structures in the respiratory tract that are damaged by smoking.	Drug that is smoked in joints.
20 pts.	?					
	A	Street name for the smokable form of cocaine.	Type of alcohol in drinks.	Poisonous gas in cigarette smoke and car exhaust fumes.	Abnormal growth of cells in the lungs.	Removal of a drug from the body that may cause unpleasant effects.
30 pts.	?					
	A	Hallucinogen, also called "angel dust."	Of hard liquor, wine, and beer, the one with the highest proof.	Black, sticky substance in tobacco that causes cancer.	Liver disease common in alcoholics.	Needing more of a drug to feel its effects.
40 pts.	?					
	A	Drug that was thought to be a cure for morphine addiction.	Gulping drinks and drinking alone.	Finely ground tobacco that is inhaled or put between the cheek and gum.	Air sacs in the lungs lose their elasticity.	Hallucinations after you've stopped using a drug.
50 pts.	?					
	A	The four methods of taking drugs.	What BAC stands for.	White spots inside the mouth that may lead to cancer.	A disease in which excessive mucus is produced in the bronchial tubes.	Glue, gasoline, butyl nitrite, etc.

Name _____

Date _____

SUBSTANCE ABUSE PREVENTION GAME ANSWER KEY (SA-78)

	DRUGS	ALCOHOL	TOBACCO	DISEASES	GENERAL
10 pts. ?	What are narcotics?	What is proof?	What is nicotine?	What are cilia?	What is marijuana?
20 pts. A	Category of drugs that come from the opium poppy.	Double the percentage of alcohol in a beverage.	Stimulant found in tobacco.	Tiny hairlike structures in the respiratory tract that are damaged by smoking.	Drug that is smoked in joints.
?	What is crack?	What is ethyl?	What is carbon monoxide?	What is lung cancer?	What is withdrawal?
A	Street name for the smokable form of cocaine.	Type of alcohol in drinks.	Poisonous gas in cigarette smoke and car exhaust fumes.	Abnormal growth of cells in the lungs.	Removal of a drug from the body that may cause unpleasant effects.
30 pts. ?	What is PCP?	What is hard liquor?	What is tar?	What is cirrhosis?	What is tolerance?
A	Hallucinogen, also called "angel dust."	Of hard liquor, wine, and beer, the one with the highest proof.	Black, sticky substance in tobacco that causes cancer.	Liver disease common in alcoholics.	Needing more of a drug to feel its effects.
40 pts. ?	What is heroin?	What are signs of alcoholism?	What is snuff?	What is emphysema?	What are flashbacks?
A	Drug that was thought to be a cure for morphine addiction.	Gulping drinks and drinking alone.	Finely ground tobacco that is inhaled or put between the cheek and gum.	Air sacs in the lungs lose their elasticity.	Hallucinations after you've stopped using a drug.
50 pts. ?	What are sniffing, swallowing, injecting, and smoking?	What is blood-alcohol concentration?	What is leukoplakia?	What is chronic bronchitis?	What are inhalants?
A	The four methods of taking drugs.	What BAC stands for.	White spots inside the mouth that may lead to cancer.	A disease in which excessive mucus is produced in the bronchial tubes.	Glue, gasoline, butyl nitrite, etc.

ACTIVITY 17: THERE'S NO DENYING IT!
(Understanding Denial)

Concept/ Description: The biggest roadblock to seeking help is denial that a problem with alcohol or other drugs exists.

Objective: To have students give examples of denial either in their own lives or in the lives of others.

Materials: Denial File worksheet (SA-79)

Directions:
1. Give each student a Denial File worksheet.
2. Discuss denial as a defense mechanism or coping strategy.
3. Discuss how denial can be a major roadblock in seeking treatment for addiction.
4. Have students give examples of denial that they have experienced. (Some may wish to keep it on a very low-key level, while others may give more personal examples.)
5. Discuss.

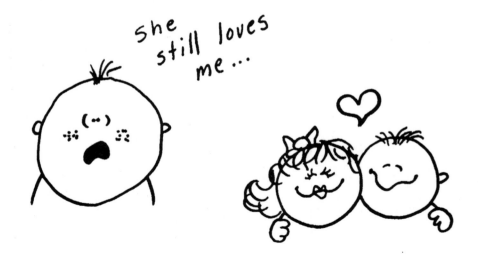

DENIAL FILE (SA-79)

DIRECTIONS: Read the definition of denial and the examples given. Give examples of denial that you have experienced, either personally or in your dealings with others.

DENIAL:

Refusal to recognize a painful or disturbing emotion or problem; ignoring a problem by acting as if it doesn't exist; keeping unpleasant information from conscious thought.

EXAMPLES:

1. Mary's mother dies. Mary still continues to set her place at the table each night.
2. Tom's parents are getting a divorce. Tom acts as if nothing is wrong. When asked if he is okay, Tom laughs and says it doesn't bother him.
3. Jodie is cut from the field hockey team. She tells her friends that she is glad and didn't really want to play anyway.
4. Jeff's girlfriend broke up with him last year and has been dating someone else. Jeff still continues to talk about her as his girlfriend.
5. Sharon drinks heavily. Last week she lost her job because she overslept after a drinking binge. Sharon blames it on her parents, who should have called her on the phone to wake her.

YOUR EXAMPLES:

_____

_____

_____

_____

_____

_____

_____

_____

ACTIVITY 18: HELP ME! I'VE FALLEN AND I CAN'T GET UP! (Seeking Help)

Concept/ Description: Alcoholics or drug addicts must first acknowledge the fact that they have a problem before they can be helped. Once the addict has recognized the problem, there are many options available.

Objective: To have students explore the various sources of help for problems with alcohol and other drugs and to compile a directory of those sources.

Materials: Directory of Resources worksheet (SA-80)
Phone books

Directions:
1. Give groups of students phone books. These can be obtained from your local phone company, or you can reproduce the self-help section and pass out copies to the students.
2. Have the groups write down local, state, and national hotlines for alcohol and other drug abuse.
3. Compile lists of agencies that treat addiction, such as hospitals, detoxification programs, and therapeutic communities. Call or write to some of the agencies and ask for pamphlets and other information describing the program.
4. Once the information has been accumulated, compile it into a directory for future reference.
5. Distribute copies to the school nurse, counselors, and others.

DIRECTORY OF RESOURCES (SA-80)

DIRECTIONS: On the left, list a source of help and its address and phone number. On the right, give a brief description of the source.

Alcohol and Other Drug Abuse

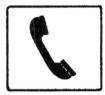

Source	Description
AL-ANON FAMILY GROUP 1-800-356-9996 BOX 862 MIDTOWN STATION NEW YORK, NY 10018	HELP FOR FAMILY AND FRIENDS OF PROBLEM DRINKERS.

ANSWER KEYS TO REPRODUCIBLES

ALCOHOL PRE-TEST (SA-1)

DIRECTIONS: Place a *T* for True or an *F* for False in the blank to the left.

F   1. Beer is "weaker" than rum or vodka.

F   2. Alcohol is digested the same way food is digested in the body.

F   3. Because alcohol is a stimulant, it tends to pep you up.

T   4. The liver is the organ responsible for "burning up" the alcohol in the body.

F   5. The body can eliminate about 5 ounces of alcohol per hour.

F   6. BAC or BAL refers to the amount of calories in an alcoholic beverage.

F   7. Black coffee and a cold shower can help to sober you up.

T   8. It is possible to die from an overdose of alcohol.

T   9. Alcohol does the greatest damage to the liver, brain, and heart.

T   10. Alcohol is high in calories and has no nutritional value.

©1993 by The Center for Applied Research in Education

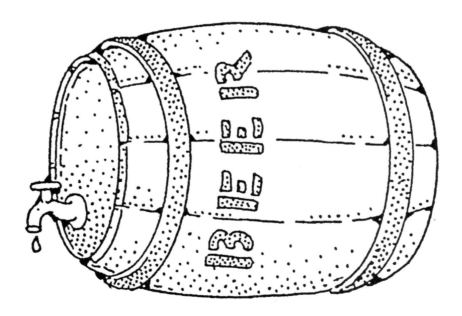

WHAT'S IN A DRINK? (SA-2)

DIRECTIONS: Find out the percentage of alcohol, plus the other ingredients in the beverages below and place the information in the blanks. Remember: a 5 oz. glass of wine, a 12 oz. can of beer, and a 1½ oz. shot of hard liquor all have the same amount of alcohol.

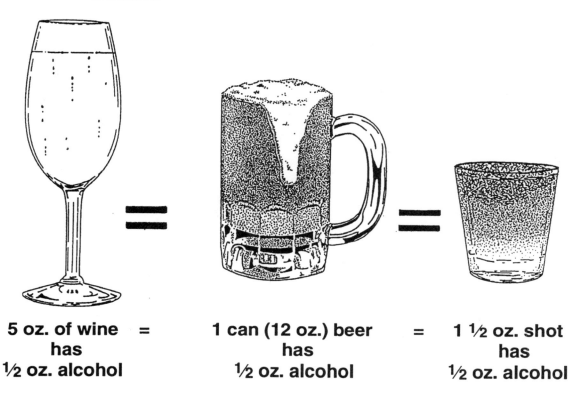

5 oz. of wine = 1 can (12 oz.) beer = 1 ½ oz. shot
has   has   has
½ oz. alcohol   ½ oz. alcohol   ½ oz. alcohol

INGREDIENTS:

Beer: _____**3–8**_____ % of alcohol, plus **fermentation of cereal grains plus malt. Hops may be**

added for flavor.

_____

_____

Wine: _____**8–14**_____ % of alcohol, plus **fermentation of grapes or other fruit.**

_____

_____

Hard liquor: _____**40–50**_____ % of alcohol, plus **distillation of a fermented brew of grain, fruit, or**

molasses.

_____

PROOF IT!! (SA-3)

Proof indicates the concentration of alcohol in a beverage. The amount of alcohol is determined by dividing the proof number in half. The higher the proof, the stronger the alcohol.

DIRECTIONS: Place the PROOF or PERCENTAGE in the blank.

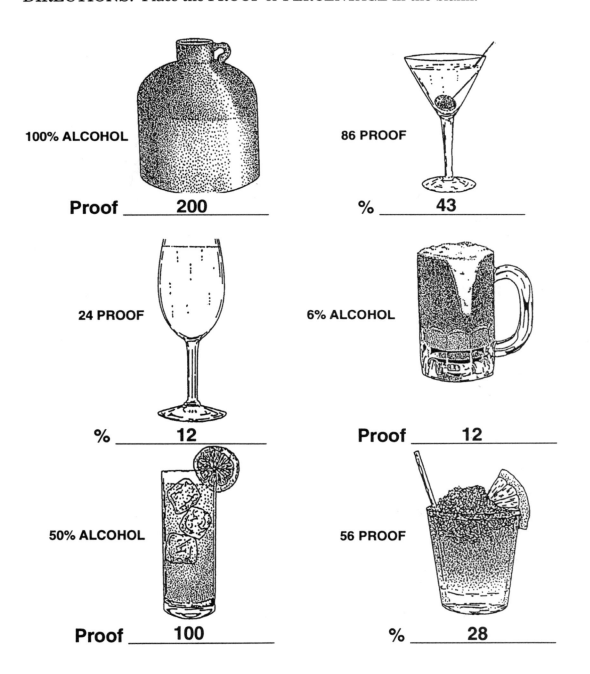

100% ALCOHOL

Proof _____ 200 _____

86 PROOF

% _____ 43 _____

24 PROOF

% _____ 12 _____

6% ALCOHOL

Proof _____ 12 _____

50% ALCOHOL

Proof _____ 100 _____

56 PROOF

% _____ 28 _____

YOU BE THE JUDGE!! (SA-7)

DIRECTIONS: Listed below are some situations involving alcohol. Decide if each action described is legal or illegal and write your decision in the blank. Find out the drinking laws for your state (contact the local police department) and check your answers.

1. A 6-year-old boy has a sip of his grandfather's beer at a family barbecue.

    legal

2. A junior high school student buys a few wine coolers.

    illegal

3. Your parents puchase a wine-making kit and make a few bottles of wine.

    legal

4. A high school student wears a T-shirt promoting beer drinking.

    legal

5. A 30-year-old woman buys a six-pack of beer from a bar on a Sunday.

    legal (if no Blue Laws)

6. A 21-year-old lends his 16-year-old brother his driver's license so he can buy alcohol.

    illegal

7. A 15-year-old girl is at a drinking party that is raided by the police. She has an open can of beer in her hand but she has not had a drink.

    illegal

8. A 22-year-old college student has a few beers at a local bar and hits a tree while driving home. His BAC is .04 percent. Is his blood-alcohol level legal or illegal?

    legal

9. A drunken man starts a fight at a movie theater and pushes a patron to the ground.

    illegal

10. A waiter serves a glass of champagne to a 17-year-old who is celebrating her birthday with her parents.

    illegal

11. A high school student "spikes" the punch at a school dance.

    illegal

12. A woman drives home from a party and is stopped by the police for weaving all over the road. She refuses to take a breathalyzer test.

    illegal

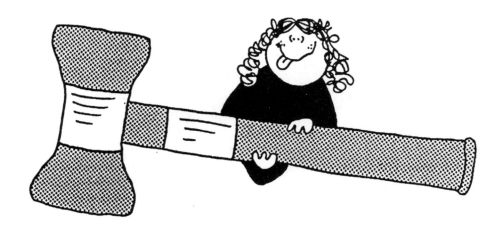

ALCOHOL CROSSWORD PUZZLE (SA-8)

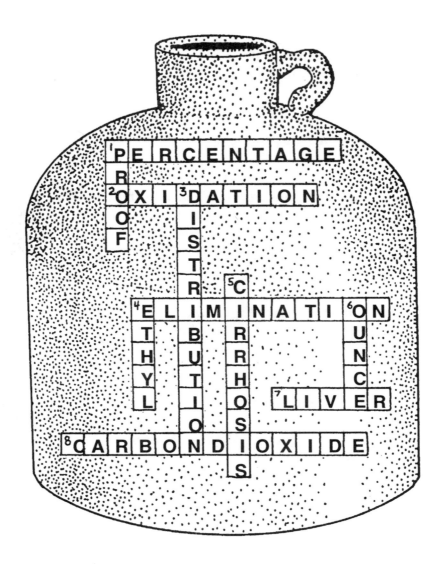

DOWN

1. Two times the percentage of alcohol in a beverage.
3. Process by which alcohol enters the bloodstream and travels to all body parts.
4. The type of alcohol used in beverages.
5. Liver disease caused by drinking heavily for many years.
6. The liver can burn up ½ _____ of alcohol per hour.

ACROSS

1. One-half of the proof.
2. Process by which the liver burns up the alcohol consumed.
4. Process by which the alcohol leaves the body.
7. Organ responsible for oxidizing alcohol.
8. During oxidation, the alcohol is changed to water, energy, and _____ (2 wds).

EFFECTS OF ALCOHOL (SA-9)

DIRECTIONS: Fill in the blanks to explain how alcohol affects a person.

HOW ALCOHOL AFFECTS A PERSON DEPENDS ON:

1. How _____**fast**_____ you drink.

2. How _____**much**_____ you drink.

3. Your body_____**weight**_____.

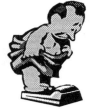

4. How much drinking you've done in the _____**past**_____.

I've been drinking for 5 years now!

5. How much _____**food**_____ is in the stomach.

6. What your _____**expectations**_____ are about drinking.

I'm gonna get loaded!!

7. _____**Where**_____ you are when you drink.

PARTY

113

EXPLODING THE MYTHS (SA-11)

DIRECTIONS: Numbered below are six myths about drinking. Below them are six correct explanations that "explode" or disprove each myth. Match each myth with its correct explanation by placing a number in the box.

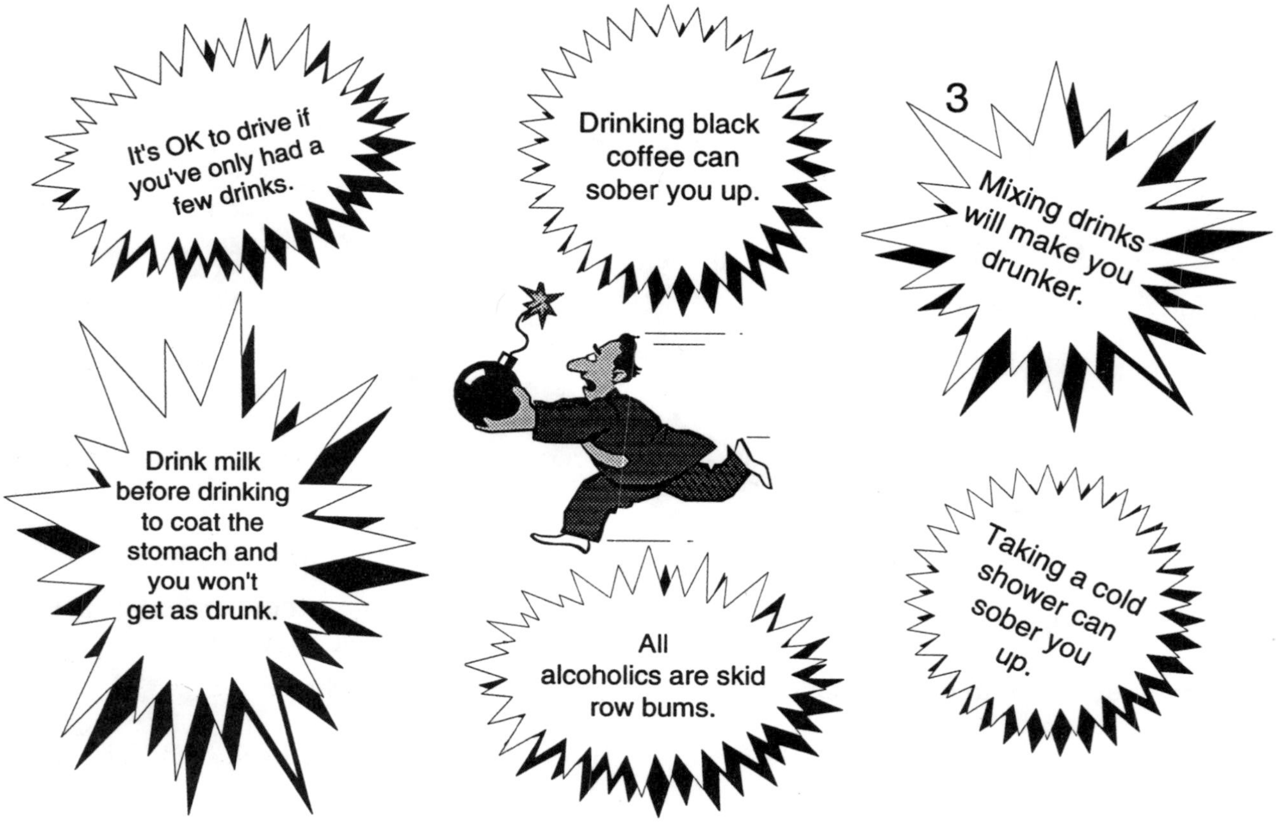

6 WRONG. The only thing you'll be is wet. Showers cannot sober you up.

2 WRONG. Drinking black coffee will make you no less drunk. Time is the only thing that can sober you up. You'll only be a wide-awake drunk.

5 WRONG. Anyone can become an alcoholic. You can be young or old, rich or poor, any race or religion.

3 WRONG. Mixing drinks may make you ill, but it's the amount that you drink that makes you drunk, not the flavor.

1 WRONG. Even a couple of drinks can impair judgement, reaction time, vision, etc.

4 WRONG. Milk and all other foods may slow down alcohol's effects, but the alcohol will still get into your bloodstream.

©1993 by The Center for Applied Research in Education

HOW MUCH DO YOU KNOW? (SA-14)

ADDICTION

DIRECTIONS: Place a *T* for True or an *F* for False in the blank to the left of each statement.

_____T_____ 1. Abuse of alcohol can lead to addiction.

_____T_____ 2. Use of alcohol and other drugs becomes the most important thing in a person's life once they are addicted.

_____F_____ 3. Alcoholism is not a disease.

_____F_____ 4. Anyone who drinks is likely to have an alcohol problem.

_____T_____ 5. After an addict has successfully stopped "using," he or she can never use alcohol or other drugs again.

_____T_____ 6. The brain and liver suffer the most damage when a person drinks heavily for many years.

_____T_____ 7. There are signs to warn a person that his or her "using" may be leading to addiction.

_____T_____ 8. When a person uses alcohol or other drugs for a long period of time, tolerance develops causing the person to need more of the substance to feel "high."

_____T_____ 9. Unpleasant physical and emotional symptoms occur when an addict tries to stop using the substance to which they are addicted.

_____T_____ 10. Drinking or using drugs when alone is a warning sign that may indicate addiction.

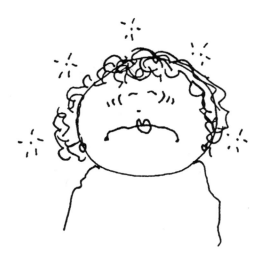

TEST YOUR SMOKING I.Q. (SA-22)

DIRECTIONS: Place a *T* for True or an *F* for False in the blank to the left.

F   1. The nicotine in cigarettes causes cancer. (Nicotine causes addiction.)

F   2. The tar in cigarettes causes addiction. (Tar causes cancer.)

T   3. Cigarette smoking can lead to heart disease.

T   4. Over 1,000 people die each day from smoking.

F   5. It is safe to smoke filtered cigarettes.

F   6. Chewing tobacco contains less nicotine than cigarettes.

T   7. Nine out of ten people with lung cancer will die.

T   8. Being in a smoke-filled room for one hour is the same as smoking one cigarette.

T   9. A woman who smokes during pregnancy can harm the fetus.

T   10. Polonium is a radioactive element found in cigarette smoke.

T   11. Cigarette smoking kills more people each year than all the deaths due to AIDS, heroin, crack, cocaine, car accidents, murder, fire, and alcohol combined.

F   12. Smoking pipes and cigars is a great deal less dangerous than smoking cigarettes.

©1993 by The Center for Applied Research in Education

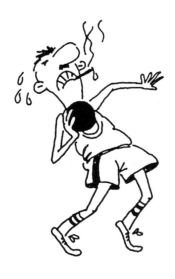

SMOKE 'N CROAK! (SA-23)

DIRECTIONS : Cigarette smoking kills more than 350,000 Americans each year. Unscramble the words and fill them into the sentence below to find out an important fact about deaths due to cigarette smoking.

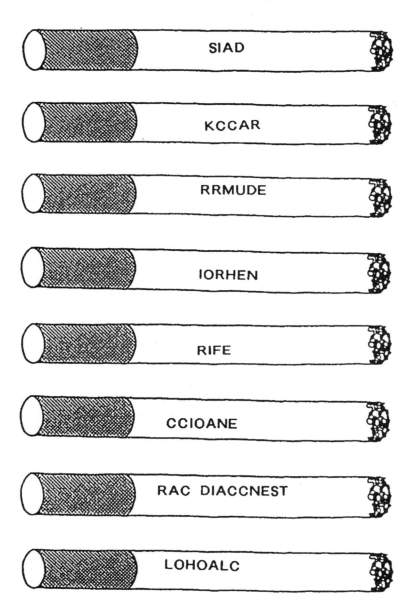

SIAD

KCCAR

RRMUDE

IORHEN

RIFE

CCIOANE

RAC DIACCNEST

LOHOALC

Cigarette smoking kills more people per year than all the deaths due to __AIDS__ , __CRACK__ ,

__MURDER__ , _HEROIN_ , __FIRE__ , __COCAINE__ , CAR ACCIDENTS , & ALCOHOL combined!

WHAT IS NICOTINE? (SA-31)

DIRECTIONS: Fill in the blanks with the correct word to make an accurate description of the drug nicotine. The pictures provide clues as to the word.

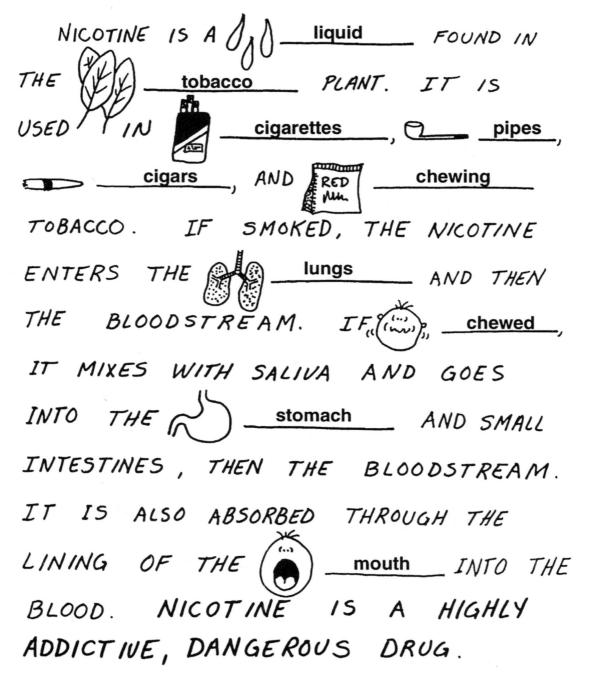

NICOTINE IS A ___liquid___ FOUND IN THE ___tobacco___ PLANT. IT IS USED IN ___cigarettes___, ___pipes___, ___cigars___, AND ___chewing___ TOBACCO. IF SMOKED, THE NICOTINE ENTERS THE ___lungs___ AND THEN THE BLOODSTREAM. IF ___chewed___, IT MIXES WITH SALIVA AND GOES INTO THE ___stomach___ AND SMALL INTESTINES, THEN THE BLOODSTREAM. IT IS ALSO ABSORBED THROUGH THE LINING OF THE ___mouth___ INTO THE BLOOD. NICOTINE IS A HIGHLY ADDICTIVE, DANGEROUS DRUG.

DON'T SMOKE!

©1993 by The Center for Applied Research in Education

SMOKING TIME LINE (SA-41)

DIRECTIONS: Write the letter of the event listed below next to the year that it occurred.

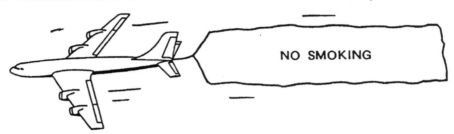

NO SMOKING

C	**1964**
F	**1965**
H	**1971**
G	**1972**
B	**1975**
D	**1983**
E	**1986**
A	**1988**

A. All U.S. airlines banned smoking on flights under two hours.

B. Minnesota passed the first state law requiring businesses, restaurants, and other institutions to establish no-smoking areas.

C. The Sureon General declared that smoking causes lung cancer, respiratory diseases, and heart disease.

D. San Francisco became the first major city to limit smoking in the workplace.

E. The Surgeon General and the National Research Council linked secondhand smoke to lung cancer and respiratory disease in nonsmokers.

F. Warning labels are required on all cigarette packages.

G. The Surgeon General issued the first report indicating that secondhand smoke is dangerous to nonsmokers.

H. Cigarette makers withdrew advertisements from television and radio.

HOW DRUGS ENTER THE BLOODSTREAM (SA-45)

DIRECTIONS: Using the words listed below, fill in the blanks to explain how drugs enter the bloodstream.

alveoli	bloodstream	muscle
stomach	capillaries	nasal
under	vein	vessels

1. **TAKEN BY MOUTH**

   The drug passes through the walls of the __**stomach**__ and then into the small

   intestine to be absorbed into the __**bloodstream**__ .

2. **INHALED**

   The drug enters the bloodstream by way of the rich supply of blood __**vessels**__ in

   the __**nasal**__ passages.

3. **SMOKED**

   The drug passes from the __**alveoli**__ (sacs) in the lungs into the __**capillaries**__
   and the bloodstream.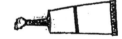

4. **APPLIED TO THE SKIN**

   The drug is applied to the skin, passes through the pores and into the tiny capillaries and
   the bloodstream.

5. **INJECTED**

   a. **Skin Popping**—the drug is injected __**under**__ the skin.

   b. **Intramuscular Injection**—the drug is injected deep into a __**muscle**__ .

   c. **Mainlining**—the drug is injected directly into a __**vein**__ .

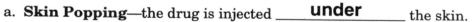

WHY PEOPLE ABUSE DRUGS (SA-46)

DIRECTIONS: Fill in the missing letters to give reasons why some people abuse drugs.

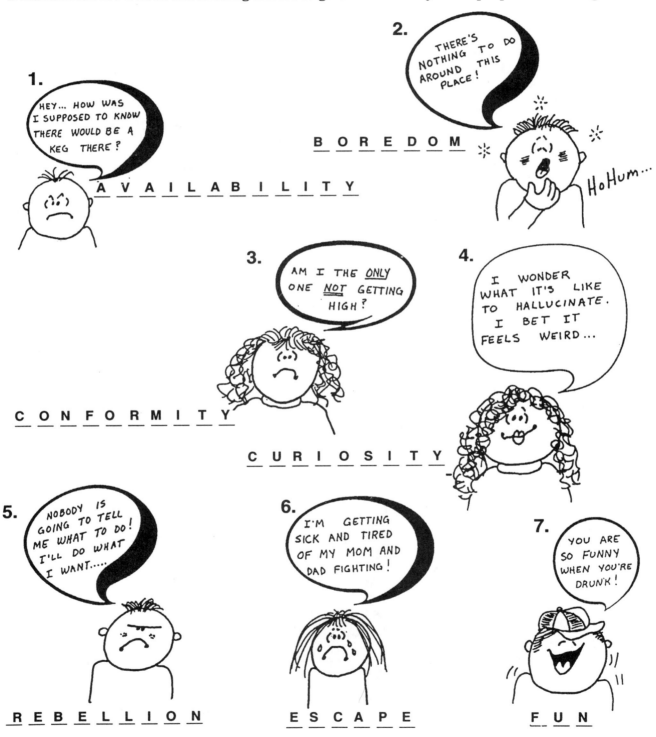

MARIJUANA PRE-TEST (SA-49)

DIRECTIONS: Place a *T* for True or an *F* for False in the blank to the left.

T____ 1. Marijuana can be eaten or smoked.

T____ 2. Though THC is the main ingredient in pot, when smoked pot produces over 2,000 chemicals.

F____ 3. THC will remain in the body for up to 12 hours. **(up to 1 month)**

T____ 4. Marijuana smoke contains more cancer-causing chemicals than cigarette smoke.

T____ 5. Marijuana is stored in the fatty tissue surrounding the reproductive organs, the lungs, and the brain.

F____ 6. The marijuana sold today is a lot weaker than that sold in the 1960s. **(a lot stronger)**

F____ 7. Marijuana used in small amounts (one joint or less) is legal.

T____ 8. Marijuana could lead to the use of other drugs.

T____ 9. The more pot you smoke, the less you need to get high. **(this is called reverse tolerance)**

F____ 10. Marijuana is legal in some states in the U.S.

©1993 by The Center for Applied Research in Education

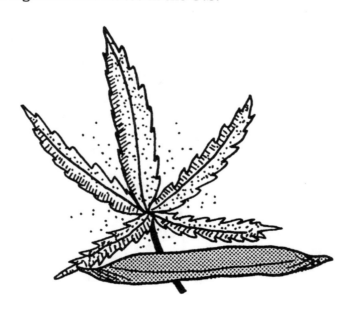

MARIJUANA (SA-52)

DRUGS:

marijuana
THC
hashish
hashish oil

DESCRIPTION:

The dried leaves, stems, and seeds of the
Cannabis sativa plant.

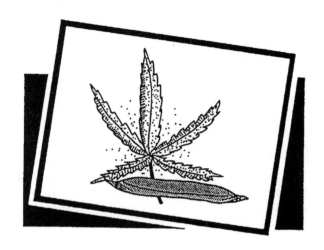

SLANG NAMES:

pot	sinsemilia	Mary Jane	Maui wowee
grass	Acapulco gold	kif	sticks
weed	Panama Red	herb	roach
reefer	Thai stick	ganga	joints
dope	Columbian		

HOW IT ENTERS THE BODY:

Smoked in joints or pipes; eaten.

EFFECTS:

increased heart rate
bloodshot eyes
dry mouth and throat
increased appetite
may impair short-term memory

altered sense of time
damaging to lungs and circulatory system
smoke contains more carcinogens than
   tobacco smoke

MEDICAL USE:

relief from side effects of cancer chemotherapy
relief from side effects of AIDS therapy
relief from symptoms of glaucoma

NARCOTICS (SA-53)

DRUGS:

heroin	Percocet
methadone	Percodan
condeine	Darvon
morphine	Talwin
opium	Demerol
Paregoric	Dilaudid

DESCRIPTION:

Powders ranging from white to dark brown; tablets, capsules, liquid. Comes from the opium poppy or is synthetic.

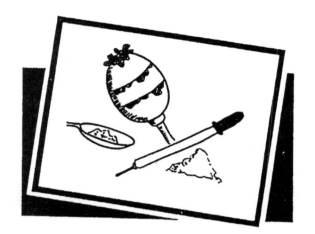

SLANG NAMES:

smack	Big H	demmies	blue velvet
horse	black tar	downtown	perkies
brown sugar	Miss Emma	dollies	Ts
junk	scag	M	
mud	schoolboy	morph	

HOW IT ENTERS THE BODY:

injected
snorted or sniffed
smoked
swallowed

EFFECTS:

euphoria followed by drowsiness, nausea, vomiting
constricted pupils
watery eyes
itching
overdose can slow breathing, cause clammy skin, convulsions, coma, death

MEDICAL USE:

pain relief
codeine: cough suppressant, pain relief
paregoric: stop diarrhea, relief from tooth pain

©1993 by The Center for Applied Research in Education

INHALANTS (SA-54)

DRUGS:

glue   nitrous oxide
nail polish remover   amyl nitrite
gasoline   butyl nitrite
aerosol sprays   liquid correction fluid
lacquer   spot remover

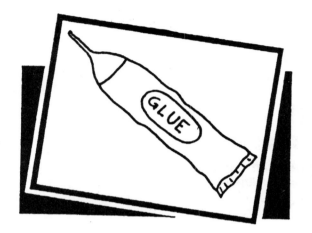

DESCRIPTION:

Dangerous fumes are concentrated in a bag, on a cloth, etc. and inhaled.

SLANG NAMES:

laughing gas   lockerroom
whippets   bullet
poppers   climax
snappers   ames
rush   bolt

HOW IT ENTERS THE BODY:

Vapors are inhaled deeply through the nose or mouth.

EFFECTS:

nausea   solvents: decrease in heart rate and breathing
sneezing, coughing   impaired judgement
nosebleeds   nitrites: rapid pulse
fatigue   headaches
lack of coordination   loss of bowel and bladder control
loss of appetite   long-term use causes hepatitis, brain damage, nervous system damage, suffocation and death

MEDICAL USE:

COCAINE (SA-55)

DRUGS:

cocaine
crack

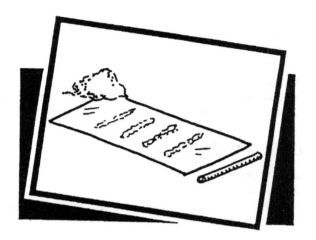

DESCRIPTION:

A white crystalline powder. Beige pellets or crystalline rocks often packaged in small vials.

SLANG NAMES:

coke	**Big C**
snow flake	**snowbirds**
white	**lady**
blow	**rock**
nose candy	**toot**

HOW IT ENTERS THE BODY:

inhaled
injected
smoked

EFFECTS:

stimulates the nervous system
dilated pupils
rise in blood pressure, heart rate, breathing, body temperature
stuffy or runny nose

insomnia
loss of appetite
paranoia
seizures
possible death from cardiac arrest

MEDICAL USE:

local anesthetic

HALLUCINOGENS (SA-56)

DRUGS:

phencyclidine
lysergic acid diethylamide (LSD)
mescaline
peyote
MDA
psilocybin

DESCRIPTION:

Drugs that distort the senses and cause
hallucinations.
Could appear as liquid, capsules, powder, blotter
paper, thin gelatin squares, mushrooms.

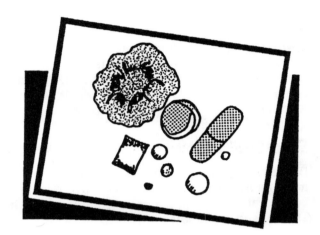

SLANG NAMES:

PCP	acid	blue heaven	buttons
angel dust	LSD	white lightning	cubes
loveboat	green dragon	sugar cubes	mesc
lovely	red dragon	microdot	blotter
hog	purple haze	window panes	shrooms
killer weed	blue cheer	super grass	scramblers

HOW IT ENTERS THE BODY:

swallowed
injected
smoked (sprayed on tobacco, marijuana, parsley)
licked off paper
chewed

EFFECTS:

time distorted
senses distorted
may produce bizarre, unpredictable behavior
person may sit for hours in a quiet dreamlike state

MEDICAL USE:

DEPRESSANTS (SA-57)

DRUGS:

barbiturates:	Nembutal, Seconal, Amytal, Tuinal, Phenobarbital
methaqualone:	Quaalude, Mequin, Parest
tranquilizers:	Valium, Librium, Thorazine
alcohol:	wine, beer, spirits

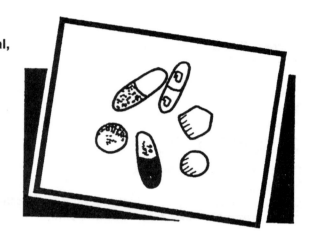

DESCRIPTION:

Drugs that depress or slow down the central nervous system and all body systems. Mixing barbiturates, methaqualone, or tranquilizers with alcohol can prove fatal.

SLANG NAMES:

yellow jackets	purple hearts	downs	booze
reds	tooeys	downers	Qs
red devils	rainbow	yellows	F-40s
red birds	ludes	sopors	
blues	714s	D	
blue heaven	barbs	phennies	

HOW IT ENTERS THE BODY:

swallowed

EFFECTS:

similar to the effects alcohol produces
small doses: calmness, relaxed muscles
larger doses: slurred speech, staggering, impaired judgement, impaired coordination
very large doses: respiratory depression, coma, death

MEDICAL USE:

to stop convulsions
relief of tension, anxiety
to induce sleep
to reduce the symptoms of alcohol withdrawal

STIMULANTS (SA-58)

DRUGS:

amphetamines: **Benzedrine, Dexedrine, Methadrine**
Ritalin
Voranil
Tepanil
Cylert
caffeine
nicotine

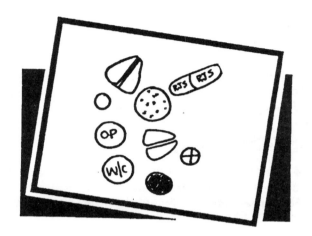

DESCRIPTION:

Drugs which cause the body systems to speed up.

SLANG NAMES:

speed	bumble bees	Christmas trees
uppers	hearts	meth
ups	footballs	copilots
crank	dexies	black beauties
pep pills		

HOW IT ENTERS THE BODY:

swallowed
snorted
injected

EFFECTS:

increased heart rate and breathing
increased blood pressure
dilated pupils
decreased appetite
dry mouth
may experience: dizziness, sweating, headache, blurred vision, sleeplessness, anxiety, moodiness
very high doses: irregular heartbeat, tremors, high fever, heart failure

MEDICAL USE:

to treat hyperactive children
to treat narcolepsy
weight control

ANABOLIC STEROIDS (SA-59)

DRUGS:
Synthetic HGH

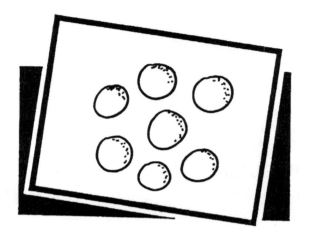

DESCRIPTION:
Powerful compounds that are similar to the male sex hormone, testosterone. These drugs are taken to increase muscle mass and strength.

SLANG NAMES:
HGH
roids

HOW IT ENTERS THE BODY:
swallowed: tablet, capsule
intramuscular injection

EFFECTS:
may initially increase muscle mass, body strength, and weight
jaundice
purple or red spots on body
swelling of feet and legs
unpleasant breath odor
depression
increased risk of heart attack, stroke, liver cancer
acne
males: sterility, withered testicles, impotence
females: irreversible masculine traits, breast reduction, sterility

MEDICAL USE:
seldom prescribed except for certain types of anemia
severe burns
some types of breast cancer

DRUG VOCABULARY CROSSWORD (SA-60)

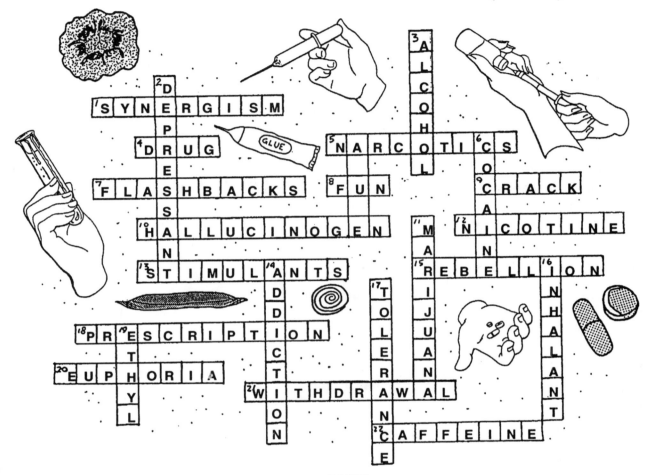

ACROSS

1. Two drugs combine to produce effects much greater than if each was used alone.
4. Any substance that chemically affects the mind or body.
5. Drugs that are derived from the opium poppy.
7. Hallucinations that occur days, weeks, and months after the drug has been used.
8. A potent form of cocaine sold in ready-to-smoke rocks.
9. A reason for using drugs.
10. Drug that causes the mind to see or imagine things that aren't real.
12. An addictive stimulant found in tobacco.
13. Drugs that speed up body systems.
15. Going against authority; a reason to use drugs.
18. Instructions by a doctor to a pharmacist.
20. Feeling of lightheadedness or being "high."
21. Removal of a drug from the body systems. This often causes physical or psychological distress.
22. A stimulant found in tea, cola, chocolate, and coffee.

DOWN

2. A type of drug that slows down body systems.
3. The most abused substance in the United States.
6. An expensive white powder that comes from the leaves of the coca bush.
11. A drug that is smoked or eaten and is also called pot, weed, and grass.
14. Needing a drug in order to survive.
16. Substance that is sniffed in order to get "high" from the fumes.
17. Needing more and more of a drug to feel its effects.
19. The type of alcohol used in beverages.

TYPES OF DRUG ABUSE (SA-62)

THE EXPERIMENTER

1. ___Curiosity___ is a motivator.

2. The user is learning about the ___mood swings___ brought on by the drug.

3. The user is learning to ___trust___ / ___mistrust___ the drug and its effects.

4. Getting ___"high"___ is a new feeling not in the normal range of emotions.

5. The user can still ___relate___ to people.

REGULAR USER

1. The decision to ___use___ has been made.

2. The user now seeks the ___"high"___ .

3. There is increased ___comfort___ and ___confidence___ in the use of the drug.

4. The ___peer___ group that the person hangs out with uses.

5. Getting "high" is more ___important___ now.

6. ___Tolerance___ develops.

7. The person becomes ___cocky___ .

8. The user has some problems ___relating___ to others.

TYPES OF DRUG ABUSE (*continued*) (SA-63)

PREOCCUPIED USER

1. The user is ____thinking____ more about drugs.

2. The user wants to be "high" ____often____.

3. ____Blackouts____ start to occur.

4. Relationships are ____difficult____.

5. The person clearly wants to ____use____ ____the____ ____drug____.

6. The person uses when ____alone____, which is very dangerous.

7. The user still thinks he or she has ____control____.

THE ADDICT

1. The addict can ____no____ ____longer____ get "high."

2. The user must take the drug to ____survive____.

3. There is no ____choice____ : you must use.

4. The person relates to ____drugs____ ,

   not to ____people____.

5. The addict will use ____any____ ____time____.

6. The behavior is both obnoxious and ____intimidating____.

7. ____Drugs____ are the user's life.

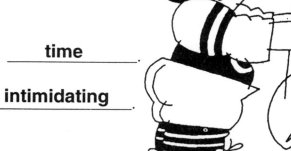

I THOUGHT I HAD THAT...

VOCAB-A-MANIA (SA-68)

DIRECTIONS: Match the word with its definition and place the correct letter in the blank to the left.

d	1.	emphysema
j	2.	caffeine
q	3.	blackout
b	4.	anabolic steroids
l	5.	tolerance
v	6.	reverse tolerance
o	7.	seizure
u	8.	judgment
t	9.	HGH
s	10.	hallucination
r	11.	euphoria
e	12.	ethyl
h	13.	cirrhosis
k	14.	paranoia
p	15.	BAC
g	16.	PCP
n	17.	tar
f	18.	nicotine
i	19.	carbon monoxide
c	20.	ice
m	21.	withdrawal
a	22.	addiction

a. compulsive use of a drug which causes physical and psychological dependence

b. synthetic hormones used by some athletes to increase muscle mass

c. a highly addictive, smokable form of "speed"

d. a disease of the lungs often caused by smoking

e. type of alcohol in alcoholic beverages

f. the ingredient in tobacco that causes addiction

g. phencyclidine, "angel dust," a potent hallucinogen

h. a liver disease that is often the result of drinking heavily for many years

i. a poisonous gas found in cigarette smoke

j. the stimulant found in coffee, tea, chocolate, and colas

k. excessive and irrational distrust of others sometimes brought on by certain types of drugs

l. needing more and more of a substance to feel its effects

m. unpleasant physical and psychological symptoms brought on by discontinuing the use of a drug

n. the ingredient in tobacco that causes cancer

o. an abnormal, violent contraction of muscles, or a convulsion sometimes due to drug use

p. the amount of alcohol in the bloodstream

q. loss of memory without passing out

r. elation or feeling of extreme well-being

s. sensory distortion

t. human growth hormone

u. the ability to form an opinion or make an evaluation

v. needing less of a drug to feel "high"

A TALE OF WOE (SA-69)

DIRECTIONS: Correct the story below by writing the correct word or words above the underlined word.

Fast Eddie, an internationally known drug dealer, had a rough

day out on the street. The wanted criminal had a kilo of heroin

2.2   **narcotic**

stolen from his car—that's 5.2 pounds of the stimulant that

opium poppy

comes from the coca bush! When Fast Eddie went to the police,

they were far from sympathetic, in fact they arrested him on

the spot. It seems they discovered crack in his pocket. Crack is

cocaine

a smokable form of glue. Fast Eddie also had too much to drink.

The police gave him a breathalyzer test which measures the

alcohol   **bloodstream**

amount of nicotine in the urine and found his BAC to be .20

percent, which is legally intoxicated.

Fast Eddie was sent to jail, but that didn't stop him. He sat

marijuana

down and lit up a joint, which is a cigarette containing opium.

The police officer in charge stopped him immediately. She

suggested that Fast Eddie join a support group such as NA

Narcotics

which stands for Nutrition Anonymous. Eddie promised to do

that as soon as he got out of jail.

Two years later Fast Eddie was released and, as promised,

joined NA and is now recovering. In fact, Eddie hasn't touched

alcohol or other drugs at all. He said the hardest part of recovery

withdrawal

was tolerance, which is when the drug is removed from the body

systems. Eddie has a long road ahead of him, but Eddie is doing

much better and is happy to be drug and alcohol free.

©1993 by The Center for Applied Research in Education

Here's a little help...

NARCOTICS
withdrawal
alcohol
2.2
opium poppy
depressant
3.5
marijuana
cocaine
synergism
bloodstream
narcotic
hallucinogen

135

OH BABY! 1 (SA-72)

DIRECTIONS: Place the words given below into the story to explain how drugs can affect the fetus.

COCAINE

seizures	premature	SIDS	kidneys
miscarriages	stillbirths	placenta	retards
	withdrawal	shock	

The use of cocaine by women in the early months of pregnancy can cause **miscarriages** or **stillbirths** . In later months, it may cause **premature** delivery.

Cocaine **retards** fetal growth and head size, and can cause malformed **kidneys** and genitals. Cocaine increases the risk of **SIDS** , Sudden Infant Death Syndrome. It may cause premature separation of the **placenta** from the uterus resulting in heavy bleeding and **shock** . Many cocaine babies are born going through **withdrawal** and suffering **seizures** .

MARIJUANA

length	fat	tremors	longer
THC	weight	visual	

The use of marijuana during pregnancy can result in low birth **length** and **weight** . **THC** , the active ingredient in marijuana, remains in the fetal brain **longer** than in the mother's brain because the fetus's brain has a higher **fat** content. Marijuana use can cause the baby to have **tremors** at birth, seizures, and **visual** problems.

136

©1993 by The Center for Applied Research in Education

OH BABY! 2 (SA-73)

ALCOHOL

facial	sex organs	Fetal Alcohol Syndrome
hyperactivity	no safe level	sleep
retardation	heart	below-normal

Alcohol use can cause **Fetal Alcohol Syndrome** (FAS), which is characterized by retarded fetal growth and infants who are born with **below-normal** weight and size. FAS includes **facial** deformity: small head, narrow eyes, flat nose, thin upper lip. Alcohol can also cause defects and deformity of the **heart**, kidneys, muscles, joints, and **sex organs**. It can cause mental **retardation**, learning disorders, **hyperactivity**, lack of coordination, and **sleep** disturbances. There is **no safe level** of use during pregnancy.

TOBACCO

six	heart	bloodstream	oxygen
increases	chemicals	lung	death
	smoke	most	

Tobacco **smoke** contains thousands of different **chemicals** that cross the placenta and enter the fetus's **bloodstream**. As a result, the amount of **oxygen** to the fetus is reduced and the risk of miscarriage increases. The chance of infant **death** in the first year also **increases**. Other negative effects include low birth weight, delivery problems, and a higher chance of infant **heart** and **lung** disease. Tobacco is the **most** damaging in the last **six** months of pregnancy.